Screening for
Brain Impairment

Second Edition

Richard A. Berg, PhD, was trained in clinical neuropsychology at the University of Houston and completed a postdoctoral fellowship in neuropsychology at the University of Nebraska Medical Center. Dr. Berg formerly worked at the St. Jude Children's Research Hospital in Memphis and was the director of the Psychology Department for Tri-State Regional Rehabilitation Hospital in Evansville, Indiana. He now works at Wilmington Health Associates, PA, Wilmington, NC. He has published widely in the field of clinical neuropsychology, and is actively involved in ongoing research.

Michael Franzen, PhD, was trained in clinical psychology at Southern Illinois University and completed a clinical internship and a postdoctoral year of training in clinical neuropsychology at the University of Nebraska Medical Center. Dr. Franzen is currently director of neuropsychology for the West Virginia University School of Medicine in Morgantown, and he serves as director of psychological training and research at Allegheny General Hospital in Pittsburgh. He has published widely in the field of clinical neuropsychology, and is actively involved in ongoing research.

Danny Wedding, PhD, received his doctorate in clinical psychology from the University of Hawaii and completed his internship on the neuropsychology service of Hawaii State Hospital. He did a subsequent year of training in neuropsychology and behavioral medicine at the University of Mississippi Medical Center. Dr. Wedding currently directs The Missouri Institute of Mental Health in St. Louis, Missouri. He has published widely in the field of clinical neuropsychology, and is actively involved in ongoing research.

Screening for Brain Impairment

Second Edition

A Manual for Mental Health Practice

Richard A. Berg, PhD
Michael Franzen, PhD
Danny Wedding, PhD

Springer Publishing Company
New York

First edition published, 1987

Springer Publishing Company, Inc.
536 Broadway
New York, NY 10012

Cover design by Holly Block
Production Editor: Joyce Noulas

94 95 96 97 98 / 5 4 3 2 1

Library of Congress Cataloging-in-Publication Data

Berg, Richard (Richard A.)
    Screening for brain impairment : a manual for mental health
practice / Richard A. Berg, Michael Franzen, Danny Wedding.—2nd
ed.
      p. cm.
    Includes bibliographical references and index.
    ISBN 0-8261-5741-6
    1. Neuropsychological tests—Handbooks, manuals, etc. 2. Brain—
Diseases—Diagnosis—Handbooks, manuals, etc. I. Franzen, Michael
D., 1954– . II. Wedding, Danny. III. Title.
    [DNLM: 1. Neuropsychology—methods. 2. Cerebral Cortex—
physiopathology. 3. Neuropsychological Tests. WL 103 B493s 1994]
RC386.6.N48B47 1994
616.8'0475—dc20
DNLM/DLC
for Library of Congress   94–10173
                                              CIP

Printed in the United States of America

To our families

Contents

Preface

This book originally was, and still is, intended for the general clinician who is faced with the task of assessing clients who may or may not have organic impairment. It is not intended to provide the expertise needed to allow general clinicians to perform neurological or neuropsychological evaluations. Both of these evaluations require specialized didactic and experiential training that takes several years to acquire and that cannot be replaced by reading this or any other book.

This book's authors are clinical psychologists with graduate training in behavioral medicine and additional specialized postdoctoral training in clinical neuropsychology. However, we are often called on to consult general clinicians who have to evaluate patients or clients whose problems may have questionable organic etiologies. It became apparent to us that there is a gap in the training of general clinicians, who are often not taught to recognize when referral to a specialist is appropriate.

We have been asked to give workshops on procedures that can be used to facilitate decision making about referrals. Evaluation by a specialist, either a neurologist or a neuropsychologist, is an expensive endeavor in terms of both money and time. Additionally, because the field of clinical neuropsychology is in a nascent state, there are certain geographical areas where individuals may not have easy access to a specialist. There is, therefore, a particular need for a set of procedures that can be used by the general clinician and that can focus the available information before a decision to refer is made.

Because this text was originally written several years ago, there has been a proliferation of new and updated assessment devices. We have made changes to reflect these new devices as well as eliminate some of the older, less useful ones for which little new data have emerged. Sections on new issues, such as acquired immunodeficiency syndrome (AIDS) and related cognitive disorders, have been added as well.

The primary goal of this book is to provide the clinician with procedures that can be used in the general outpatient clinical setting. For the most part, the procedures described in this book can be used with a minimal investment in equipment.

A second goal of this book is to provide the general clinician with a translation of those terms and activities that are used by the specialist. The specialist has his own vocabulary, which can be useful when discussing conditions with other specialists but which obfuscates the issues for the general clinician. Unfortunately, there is no certain method for ensuring that every specialist's report is written with plain diction and in behavioral rather than "foreign" terms. However, if the general clinician is armed with some knowledge of the language of specialists, she can derive more benefit for the referral report. The glossary that is provided at the end of this book should help the reader become more familiar with many of the technical terms and much of the jargon found in neurology and neuropsychology.

Not all of the procedures described in this book should be used with every patient. However, the procedures described here provide a useful outline for the evaluation of the patient with suspected central nervous system dysfunction. The first step is always to take a thorough history. The depth of history will vary from patient to patient. If information regarding the etiology of an organic problem surfaces during the history interview, that area should be followed up with a more intensive line of questioning. Of course, the direction pursued by the clinician taking the history will be determined in part by some understanding of the way in which various neurological disorders present clinically and across time. We will attempt to present this information succinctly in the first two chapters of this book.

If the history, clinical presentation, or referral of a patient suggests an organic etiology, then a Mental Status Examination (MSE) should be conducted. The procedures in the chapter on the MSE can be used as a flexible guide to evaluation. The purpose of the MSE is to uncover additional information before a decision to refer is made. In no case should a MSE take the place of the complete neuropsychological and neurological evaluation.

There are three possible outcomes of the MSE. First, the MSE may not result in any indications of organic etiology, in which case no referral is made. Second, the MSE may uncover some definite evidence of organic impairment, and the general clinician may decide to refer to a specialist.

Third, the MSE may uncover only suggestions of impairment, in which case the general clinician may want to investigate further the possibility of organic impairment before referring to a specialist. The chapters on screening instruments can be useful at this point. For example, if the history and MSE uncover suspected deficits in visual functioning, the general clinician can turn to the chapter on screening test for perceptual and motor functions. On the basis of the patient's performance, a better decision to refer can be made.

There is yet another source of information that the clinician can use in deciding whether or not to refer, and that is the specialist herself. Oftentimes the needed information is only a telephone call away. If the case does not involve an emergent condition, it would be better to send a copy of the MSE or screening results to the specialist. Naturally, these materials should not be sent without advance warning. The best situation would be one in which the general clinician has developed a working relationship with the specialist. We would also recommend that the general clinician be consumer-minded in the search for a specialist. Not all specialists are equal in skill or in the ability to provide useful information to the original referral source. The general clinician can give feedback to the specialist regarding the utility of the results and report and can ask further questions that have not been addressed by the report. The specialist can be helped by being provided a complete history, along with a copy of the results of any evaluations conducted prior to referral. It also facilitates the process if the general clinician can provide a specific question in the referral request.

We hope this book will be useful to the general clinician. We believe it will prove helpful to both the practicing clinician and to graduate students, who can use it to learn more about cortical dysfunctions and to increase their personal repertoires of assessment techniques. Ultimately, we hope the book will lead to more accurate assessment and better treatment for the large number of patients who will be screened by clinicians who have read this book.

The feedback we have received on the book since the original publication has been gratifying and indicates that our original goals of providing a useful resource for general clinicians and students have, in large measure, been met. We hope that this updated version will continue to prove to be a useful adjunct for clinicians.

Acknowledgments

A number of people have helped us plan, develop, and communicate the ideas in this book. We are, of course, appreciative of our teachers, and we hope our own students learn as much from us. We also appreciate the help of our colleagues who have taken time to discuss the general issues presented in this volume. These include John Linton, Johnnie L. Gallemore, Raymond J. Corsini, and Leon McGahee, all of whom have contributed in different ways to this text and to our own professional growth. We very much appreciate the creative efforts of Carol Stroud, who produced much of the artwork without compensation and without complaining. Barbara Cubic, Piera Bortolini, Ann Holly, and Kelly Webster-Kelly did much of the typing and attended to an endless number of details. Cynthia Wedding and Cynthia Berg also helped us in numerous ways during the months devoted to researching and preparing this book. Finally, we wish to acknowledge the support and contribution of our parents and our extended families. It is to them that this book is dedicated.

1
Neurological Disorders

Psychologists and other nonmedical mental health personnel routinely evaluate patients with psychiatric disorders. However, oftentimes psychiatric disorders coexist with neurological disorders; at other times neurological disorders may present with classic psychiatric symptoms. Although neuropsychologists and psychiatrists are typically trained in differential diagnosis of these two classes of disorders, other mental health workers without special interests in brain functions often receive little or no training in how to assess the probability of brain disorders. They may be unaware of classic signs that signal cognitive impairment and indicate the need for referral to neurologists or other competent medical authorities.

In this chapter we survey traditional neurodiagnostic categories, presenting what we believe to be the most essential facts that need to be remembered by all mental health personnel. We also review the types of neurodiagnostic data likely to be included in a patient's chart, so that the reader will be able to read and understand this sometimes cryptic information. We discuss the relevance of the MSE and the patient's history, and, finally, we review the major screening techniques readily available to all psychologists to help identify those patients with likely brain disease.

BRAIN TUMORS

Patients with cerebral tumors are routinely seen in the neuropsychology laboratory, and they are not uncommon in general clinical practice. All psychologists should have a basic understanding of neoplastic disease, Because *the first signs of a brain tumor are often psychological, and tumor symptoms may mimic depression or anxiety*. Depression and psychomotor slowing are commonly found to accompany cerebral impairment, and anxiety is a prominent features of tumors in and around the third ventricle (Hall, 1980).* In addition, vague mental symptoms are oftentimes the only initial complaints of the patient with a cerebral lesion. Taylor (1982) states that some perceptible cognitive deficit is present in 77% of brain tumor cases, confusion is present in 59%, and disorientation occurs in approximately 40%. Furthermore, one study found that 100% of patients with limbic system tumors were diagnosed initially as having psychiatric disease.

Limbic system tumors mimic both schizophrenia and psychotic depression. They stand as an especially striking example of the importance of a thorough differential diagnosis and underscore the importance of at least a rudimentary understanding of brain disease for every psychologist.

Since psychologists are the point of entry into the health care system for many patients, it is critical that all psychologists be sensitive to the symptoms associated with intracranial tumors. *Headaches are the most common single complaint of patients with brain tumors*, and headaches will be present in about 60% of cases. Headaches will be the first sign of brain tumor in approximately 20% of cases (Reitan & Wolfson, 1985). The clinician's suspicion is raised when the patient reports that headaches are worse on arising in the morning, that they awaken him from sleep, or that they improve as the day progresses. Headaches associated with brain tumors tend to be exacerbated by coughing, sneezing, lifting, or straining to pass stools; they are often relieved when the patient lies down. The headaches are typically described as constant and nonpulsating. The pain is likely to be lateralized if a tumor is present above the tentorium (the structure that divides the cerebrum from the cerebellum); however, if elevated intracranial pressure is present, headache pain tends to be bifrontal or bioccipital, regardless of the location of the tumor.

Any history of projectile vomiting in adults increases the likelihood of organic disease, especially when the vomiting is not preceded by nausea and when the patient's headache improves after vomiting.

Seizures occur as a first symptom of tumors in approximately 15% of

---

*The reader is encouraged to consult the glossary found at the end of this book for the meaning of any neurological or neuropsychological term that may be unfamiliar.

cases; they occur at some time in about 20% to 30% of all tumor cases (Strub & Black, 1988). The clinician should be especially suspicious when seizures develop in the adult in the absence of head trauma, alcoholism, or some obvious causal factor. Papilledema (swelling of the optic disc) is the result of increased intracranial pressure, and it can be readily observed with an ophthalmoscope. Papilledema can be an important sign of a brain tumor. While psychologists typically lack the training and equipment necessary for a detailed ocular examination, we believe psychologists should routinely examine the patient's eyes to check for ptosis, cranial nerve defects, and possible metabolic problems. In addition, we believe it is important that all patients who present with any possibility of brain disease be asked about bowel and bladder function. *The clinician should always seek medical evaluation for the patient who presents with signs of cognitive impairment in tandem with incontinence of recent onset.* Finally, any report of increased sensitivity to the effects of drugs or alcohol should alert the clinician to the possibility of a brain tumor.

The clinical presentation of neoplastic disease can also include drowsiness, impaired judgment, memory loss, and altered mental functioning. Screening measures (discussed in Chapters 6 to 10 of this book) can be especially helpful in providing data for decision making in these cases. *Although symptoms will vary according to lesion type, location, and rate of growth, at least 50% of tumor cases will involve psychiatric symptoms.* This is especially likely in the case of tumors involving the limbic system or the frontal or temporal lobes. Hallucinations may occur, along with other psychological symptoms such as depression, apathy, elation, loss of fundamental social skills, and subtle changes in personality. The general rule is that slow-growing tumors produce changes in personality and allow premorbid tendencies to become manifest; more rapidly growing tumors lead to cognitive defects; the most rapidly growing lead to acute organic reactions with obvious impairment of consciousness (Lishman, 1978). The only early signs of a tumor may be the patient's torpid mental state, a mild slowing in behavioral responsivity, mild impairment on neuropsychological measures, and a characteristically long pause before answering questions. However, the brain is an astonishingly adaptable organ, and tumors that are sufficiently slow-growing may be totally asymptomatic or may produce such subtle signs that the change will be vaguely discerned by family members but will be missed by all but the most perspicacious clinicians.

It is useful for the psychologist to be acquainted with the major methods of classifying tumors. First of all, tumors in the central nervous sys-

tem can be *primary or secondary*. Primary tumors are those that actually arise from cells within the central nervous system (CNS); secondary
tumors arise in other areas of the body and spread or metastasize
through the blood stream to the brain and other organs. Approximately
15% of intracranial tumors are metastatic; usually the original host site
is the lung or the breast (Wiederhdt, 1982). A total of 18% of patients
who die from cancer will be shown at autopsy to have intracranial metastases (Adams & Victor, 1977). The prognosis for the patient with
metastatic cancer is uniformly bleak, and patients who develop brain
metastases typically live for only a few months. Neuropsychological
evaluation of the patient with secondary brain metastatic lesions
presents a spotty picture of weaknesses, with multiple pockets of dysfunction across the hemispheres.

Tumors are also sometimes classified as *intrinsic or extrinsic*. Intrinsic tumors develop from support cells within neural tissue; extrinsic tumors develop outside the brain, typically in the meninges. The most
common example is the meningioma, a tumor that is usually slow-growing, developing between the skull and the brain. About 20% of intracranial tumors are meningiomas. They are easily identified with brain scans
or computerized tomography, and they can usually be surgically re-
sected. If the tumor is identified in time, the patient's prognosis is good.
Mental functions are affected by the pressure exerted by the space-occu-
pying properties of the meningioma, and sometimes by erosion of the
surrounding neural tissue. Neuropsychologically, the meningioma
presents a less lateralized picture, and it rarely produces suppressions.
(Suppressions refer to the failure to perceive a stimulus on one side with
bilateral simultaneous stimulation. Suppressions can be auditory, visual,
or tactile, and are commonly seen with intrinsic tumors.) In addition, in
the case of meningiomas, the psychologist is less likely to observe the
striking differences between verbal and performance IQ values that are
common with intrinsic tumors. Middle-aged women appear to be at especially high risk for developing meningiomas (Bubb, 1984).

Brain tumors can be classified as *benign or malignant*, depending on
the rapidity of growth of the tumor and the likelihood of spread to surrounding tissue. About 40% of brain tumors are benign; however, this
distinction is of less value in the case of neural neoplasms insofar as any
tumor that invades the cranial vault is dangerous and potentially lethal.
Lethality is rated on a graduated scale, with Grade I neoplasms the least
dangerous and Grade IV neoplasms the most dangerous.

Finally, tumors can be meaningfully classified by type according to
the nature of the original cell from which they derive. Gliomas, for ex-

ample, arise from glial cells, the connective tissue of the brain. Gliomas are the most common form of brain tumor and comprise approximately 50% of intracranial tumors. These are often lethal tumors, and approximately 75% of patients with gliomas will die within 12 months of diagnosis, no matter what the treatment (Parsons, 1983). Subtypes of gliomas include the highly lethal glioblastoma multiforme, astrocytomas, ependymomas, oligodendrogliomas, and medulloblastomas. The glioblastoma multiforme is the most common form, comprising about 50% of gliomas. These lesions occur most frequently in men between the ages of 40 and 60. Because most cases of glioblastoma develop from astrocytes, some writers refer to glioblastomas as astrocytomas, Grade III or IV.

In general, children are more likely to develop tumors arising in the *brainstem and cerebellum*, whereas primary tumors in the cerebral cortex are more common in adults. The clinical presentation of tumors is more variable in children, and it is more difficult to predict how a neoplasm will affect function in the developing brain. Even in the adult, because localization of some lesions may be difficult, since bilateral or diffuse dysfunction can result from pressure effects and edema.

VASCULAR DISORDERS

Blood supplies the brain with oxygen and glucose and disposes of heat and metabolic wastes; disruption of regular blood flow to specific brain areas for more than a few minutes will almost always result in damage to the neural tissue surrounding the damaged vessel. Fortunately, there is redundancy in the complexity of cerebral vascularity, and collateral circulation can often provide blood to a region of the brain when it is cut off from its normal supply.

Cerebrovascular accidents (CVAs), also referred to as apoplexy or strokes, represent a public health problem of enormous proportions. CVAs are the third leading cause of death in the United States, and it is the rare individual whose life or family has not been affected in some way by vascular disease. Approximately 250, 000 people suffer strokes each year in the United States; of these, 10% will die immediately, and 20% to 40% will die in the months following their strokes. Of the survivors, 10% will be totally disabled and will have to be institutionalized, 40% will require nursing care, 40% will have a persistent, mild neurological defect, and only 10% will totally recover (Wiederhold, 1982). For those who do recover, *improvement will typically follow a deceler-*

*ating learning curve, with the most improvement noted in the first 6
months and with physical disabilities typically resolving more quickly
than cognitive defects.*

The occurrence of a cerebrovascular accident is almost always preceded by the process of atherosclerosis, in which arteries become hard-
ened and clotted with yellowish-white layers of cholesterol. This gradual stenosis (progressive narrowing of the cerebral vessels) at some point
may totally occlude blood flow. Carotid endarterectomy, a surgical technique for cleaning the vessels carrying blood to the brain, is sometimes
helpful in reestablishing blood supply.

Epidemiological research has isolated the major risk factors for stroke.
Increasing age and hypertension stand alone as the two best individual
predictors of cerebrovascular disease. Systolic pressure is a slightly better predictor than diastolic. However, atherosclerosis, diabetes, rheu-
matic heart disease, smoking, and use of birth control pills are also major predictors, as are race and sex (African-Americans have more strokes
than whites, and men have more strokes than women). In addition, a
person with a history of a cerebrovascular accident is at least 10 times as
likely (as the average person of his age and sex) to have another stroke.
The process of atherosclerosis is intimately linked to behavior, habit,
and lifestyle, and it becomes increasingly clear that there is nothing "ac-
cidental" about cerebrovascular accidents.

A basic understanding of vascular anatomy is essential for understanding cerebrovascular disease. The brain is supplied bilaterally by the internal carotid arteries and by the vertebral arteries. The internal carotid divides on each side to form the anterior and middle cerebral arteries. The
vertebral arteries form a single basilar artery, which divides at the top of
the midbrain to form paired posterior cerebral arteries. The posterior cerebral arteries, which supply the thalamus, the occipital lobes, and the
medial temporal lobes. The entire system is linked by the Circle of Willis
and by the anterior and posterior communicating arteries, providing for
collateral circulation.

Most strokes occur in the region of the middle cerebral artery (see
Figure 1.1). This region serves major motor and sensory areas around
the Rolandic fissure, accounting for the paralysis and sensory deficits
that often accompany a stroke. A stroke in the middle cerebral artery is
likely to produce contralateral weakness (with the arms and face weaker
than the leg), contralateral sensory loss, homonymous hemianopsia, and
dementia. If the dominant hemisphere is involved, an expressive aphasia
is likely to result. Middle cerebral artery strokes on the right side will
frequently produce denial of defects (anosognosia). Left-sided neglect is

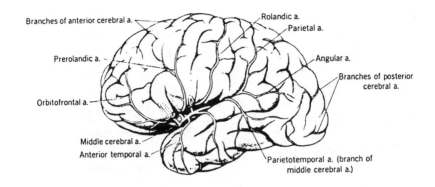

Branches of anterior cerebral a.
Rolandic a.
Parietal a.
Prerolandic a.
Angular a.
Branches of posterior cerebral a.
Orbitofrontal a.
Middle cerebral a.
Anterior temporal a.
Parietotemporal a. (branch of middle cerebral a.)

FIGURE 1.1 Lateral view of the right hemisphere illustrating the distribution of the middle cerebral artery. *Source:* Norback, C., & Demarest, R. (1981). *The human nervous system, 3rd edition*. New York: McGraw-Hill.

also common in these cases. *If the stroke affects gaze on either side, the eyes will tend to "look" toward the side of the lesion.*

Wolf (1980) has observed that total occlusion of the middle cerebral artery is more lethal in younger patients than in the elderly because in old age there has been sufficient cerebral atrophy to insure that the cerebral edema that accompanies a middle cerebral artery stroke does not cause an abrupt rise in intracranial pressure or herniation and brainstem compression.

Anterior cerebral artery infarcts are more rare than middle cerebral artery strokes and may produce contralateral weakness in the leg (while sparing the arm), contralateral sensory loss, dementia, urinary incontinence, and an affective disturbance. In addition, primitive grasp and sucking reflexes may be produced on the contralateral side.

Posterior cerebral artery infarcts are also relatively rare, but they produce fascinating clinical phenomena (see Figure 1.2). Memory impairment is often present, especially when there is temporal lobe involvement. Contralateral visual field cuts will occur with damage to the calcarine cortex. Alexia without agraphia is common when the damage is to the dominant occipital lobe along the posterior corpus callosum.

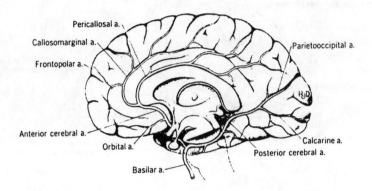

FIGURE 1.2 Midsagittal section illustrating the medial distributions of the anterior, middle, and posterior cerebral arteries. *Source:* Norback, C., & Demarest, R. (1981). *The human nervous system, 3rd edition*. New York: McGraw-Hill.

Bilateral posterior cerebral infarcts will often lead to cortical blindness with personal denial of disability. This form of anosognosia is called *Anton's syndrome*. In general, posterior strokes are far more likely to produce bilateral signs of damage. If the stroke is low enough to affect the reticular formation, loss of consciousness and eventual death will result.

Cerebrovascular accidents can be conveniently (if not precisely) categorized as either infarcts (occlusions) or hemorrhages. The former is more common by a ratio of about 3 to 1; however, the hemorrhage is a far more serious neurological event and is lethal about four times as often as the infarct (Lishman, 1978).

Infarcts or obstructive strokes can be further subdivided into thrombotic or embolic subtypes. A *thrombus* occurs as the result of the accumulation of arteriosclerotic plaques, usually at the bifurcation of a vessel. The thrombus typically develops slowly and may be preceded by transient ischemic attacks (TIAs). Hypertension, diabetes, and smoking are all important risk factors for the development of thrombotic infarcts, which typically occur during sleep, probably because of the mild state of hypotension present when the patient is supine and sleeping. Thrombotic occlusions are more common than embolic ones.

The embolus is a fatty deposit that has broken away from a blood vessel wall or, less commonly, a fragment of a thrombotic lesion that floats through the blood stream until it becomes lodged in a vessel, blocking the passage of blood and producing *ischemia*. The onset of the embolic stroke is sudden; there are no warning signs. Headache is usually absent immediately after the stroke and resolution, if it occurs, is rapid.

Hemorrhages are extremely serious neurological emergencies that result from blood spilling from a vessel and destroying surrounding brain tissue. Blood is often released under considerable pressure, and the eventual outcome of a particular stroke may be a function of whether or not blood is released away from or toward the brain itself. The onset of the hemorrhage is typically sudden and may be induced by physical exertion. Unlike thrombotic strokes, hemorrhages rarely occur during sleep. Severe headaches and loss of consciousness are the most common initial symptoms. Neuropsychological assessment of the patient who has had a cerebral hemorrhage almost always reveals suppressions and a strongly lateralized pattern of deficits.

Parsons (1983) has provided an analogy that can be used for appreciating the different varieties of traumatic hemorrhages—extradural, subdural, subarachnoid, and intracerebral. One needs first to remember that the brain is surrounded by a series of protective coverings—the meninges. At birth there are only two membranes: the pia-arachnoid, which adheres closely to the brain, and the dura, which is attached to the skull. The arachnoid eventually separates from the pia but remains connected to it by a weblike process that forms the subarachnoid space. Parsons suggests that the student imagine that the brain was sprayed with a protective coat (the pia), wrapped in a sheet of foam rubber to prevent jolting (the arachnoid), sealed in a polyethylene bag (the dura), and then suspended from the roof of a very sturdy container (the skull) by a series of threads (the veins running to the sagittal sinus). An extradural hemorrhage occurs when the outer container fractures and a skull shard ruptures a meningeal artery. Blood promptly flows into the epidural space. Patients may recover briefly following an injury of this sort, but they relapse quickly as intracranial pressure rises. The pupil on the affected side becomes dilated and fixed, and there is a contralateral hemiparesis. Immediate neurosurgical intervention is required.

The subdural hematoma is an equally serious hemorrhage that occurs following relatively minor injuries (which may be so trivial as to go either unreported or unremembered). Following the Parsons analogy, the subdural hematoma occurs when one of the veins that suspends the brain from the sagittal sinus is ruptured. Blood gradually accumulates between the dura and the arachnoid layer, and symptoms may be not develop until hours or days after the traumatic event. *The clinician who works with the elderly and with alcoholics should be sensitive to the fact that subdural hematomas are especially frequent in both of these groups and that CT scans can be normal in as many as 10 % of cases of subdural hematoma* (Parsons, 1983). It is also important to remember that chronic subdural hematomas are more likely to impair consciousness and are less likely to affect movement, sensation, or vision because most of their effect results from pressure rather than from specific neural destruction. In the patient who presents with marked clouding of consciousness or who is in a coma without severe hemiparesis, a subdural hematoma is a far more likely possibility than an ischemic stroke (Wolfe, 1980). The subarachnoid hemorrhage accounts for 5% to 10% of strokes and happens when bleeding occurs beneath the arachnoid layer. It is characterized by intense headaches and neck stiffness and by the presence of blood in the cerebrospinal fluid. The hemorrhage can result from trauma; more often it results from the bursting of an *aneurysm* (a congenital weakness in a vessel wall) or from an *arteriovenous malformation* (a congenital deformity in a vessel). The aneurysm will sometimes "balloon" and produce pressure effects. This results in an increased risk of rupturing because of the increased fragility of the vessel wall. An aneurysm that has not ruptured may be asymptomatic but will typically produce localized neuropsychological deficits, with a low Impairment Index on the Halstead-Reitan Battery (Golden, 1981). Signs of a ruptured aneurysm include nausea, vomiting, and headaches. *Berry aneurysms*, so named because of their berrylike shape, are small, thin-walled aneurysms typically found at the bifurcation of vessels.

The psychologist will not typically see patients who have hemorrhaged, at least not in the acute state, but he or she will encounter patients who are having TIAs. TIAs are temporary reductions in blood supply to the brain, which, by definition, cannot last for more than 24 hours. They do not result in the death of neural tissue, but they do produce clinical signs, and they increase the likelihood that the patient will develop more serious cerebrovascular disorders. Twenty-five to forty percent of patients with TIAs will have cerebral infarcts within five years; this incidence is 10 times that of people of the same age and sex in the general population (Olsen, Brumback, Gascon, & Christoferson, 1981).

The symptoms of a TIA will vary, depending on whether the carotid artery or the vertebrobasilar system is involved. In general, the symptoms of a TIA include vertigo, dysarthria, ataxia, vomiting, headaches, visual disturbances, motor or sensory loss, agraphia, and confusion. Although historically TIAs have been thought to produce little cognitive damage, closer analysis with neuropsychological testing reveals that mild cognitive impairment is found in these patients prior to the development of actual infarcts (Lezak, 1983).

When a vascular disorder is suspected, the clinician should always expand the history and inquire about visual disturbances and the presence of relevant risk factors, such as hypertension and oral contraceptives. In addition, the presence of crossed neurological signs (e.g., monocular blindness and contralateral hemiparesis or right-sided facial weakness with left hemiparesis) is strongly suggestive of vascular disease. It is important to appreciate that vascular disease can mimic endogenous depression; this is especially common in collagen vascular disease such as systemic lupus erythematosus (Lechtenberg, 1982). These patients will often respond to treatment with antidepressant medication.

One frequent consequence of stroke is impaired circulation of the cerebrospinal fluid (CSF). *This can produce normal pressure hydrocephalus, characterized by a classic triad of clinical signs: dementia, gait disturbance, and urinary incontinence. Any patient presenting this constellation of symptoms should be referred at once for medical, and preferably neurological, evaluation.* Treatment usually involves shunting CSF fluid from the lateral ventricles into the general circulation. Because the cause of the disorder is unknown, it is sometimes referred to as *occult hydrocephalus*. The peak age of onset is in the late fifties.

THE DEMENTIAS

The patient with a dementing illness is, in the most real and terrifying sense of the phrase, losing his mind. The term *dementia* refers to a clinical syndrome in which there is loss of brain function because of diffuse organic brain disease. It is a general term but still somewhat more precise than the vague phrase "organic brain syndrome."

The dementias are characterized by insidious onset, dysfunction that is localized primarily in the cerebral hemispheres, demonstrable patho-

TABLE 1.1   Major Causes of Dementia

Degenerative diseases of the CNS	Intracranial space-occupying lesions
Alzheimer's disease	Head trauma
Pick's disease	Epilepsy
Huntington's chorea	Infections
Parkinson's disease	Meningitis
Progressive supranuclear palsy	Encephalitis
Vascular disorder	Syphilis
Multiinfarct dementia	Creutzfeldt-Jacob disease
Arteriovenous malformation	Kuru
Carotid artery occlusive disease	Multifocal leukoencephalopathy
Subarachnoid hemorrhage	Toxins and drugs
Cerebral embolism	Alcohol
Binswanger's disease	Drugs (prescription and
Metabolic, endocrine, and nutritional	nonprescription)
disease	Heavy metals (arsenic, lead, mercury,
Hypothyroidism and hyperthyroidism	thallium)
Hypocalcemia and hypercalcemia	Carbon monoxide
Hepatic failure	Organic solvents
Wilson's disease	Miscellaneous
Renal failure	Multiple sclerosis
Dialysis encephalopathy	Muscular dystrophy
Cushing's syndrome	Normal pressure hydrocephalus
Hypopituitarism	
Electrolyte disturbances	
Wernicke-Korsakoff syndrome	
Vitamin deficiency (especially B_1, B_6,	
B_{12}, niacin, folate)	

logical changes in cerebral tissue, and the presence of memory loss as a common primary initial concern. Some writers define dementias as disorders that are irreversible; however, the more general current practice is to include a variety of conditions (e.g., Cushing's syndrome, nutritional deficiencies, Wilson's disease, etc.) that can be treated with a potential reversal of the clinical signs of dementia. Table 1.1 lists the major causes of dementia. Schamhorst (1992) has proposed a useful mnemonic for remembering the most common reversible causes of dementia. This mnemonic is listed in Table 1.2.

The problem of dementia is becoming a public health concern of unparalleled dimensions as the lifespan of the typical American continues to expand. Half of the U.S. population currently live to at least the age of 75, and one-fourth live to the age of 85. However, with increasing age each of us is at increasing risk for developing a dementing illness, since 4% to 5% of people over the age of 65 have a moderate to severe de-

TABLE 1.2   Mnemonic for Common Reversible Causes of Dementia

Drugs or alcohol use
Emotional disorders
Metabolic or endocrine disorders
Eye and ear dysfunctions
Nutritional deficiencies
Trauma, tumors, or toxins (e.g., lead poisoning)
Infections
Arteriosclerotic complications of the heart and brain

mentia. More than 50% of the patients in nursing homes carry the diagnosis of dementia, which is estimated to be the fifth leading cause of death in the United States (Lechtenberg, 1982).

Alzheimer's disease is the single most common cause of dementia, accounting for at least 65% of cases. There were less than 3 million cases of probable Alzheimer's disease in 1980, but Census Bureau projections suggest *there will be a total of 10.3 million U.S. citizens with Alzheimer's disease by the year 2050* (Evans, 1990). Caring for these patients will require prodigious resources. The *current* cost of Alzheimer's to the U.S. economy is between $80 and $90 billion (about 10% of the cost of all health care expenditures combined), and the average cost to families is about $18,000 per year (Moran, 1990). These costs are bound to increase in the future.

Onset of symptoms occurs after the age of 40 in 96% of cases and between the ages of 45 and 65 in 80% of cases (Lechtenberg, 1982). Some authors prefer to restrict the diagnosis to cases involving earlier onset (prior to the age of 65), and use the term senile dementia of the Alzheimer's type (SDAT) to refer to those cases with onset after age 65. However, there is little evidence to suggest that the two disorders are separate pathological processes. It is clear, though, that earlier onset is associated with a more severe and more rapid course than is found with cases involving later onset (Lezak, 1983).

Alzheimer's disease is a disorder that strikes females almost three times as often as males, for reasons that remain unclear (Bachman et al., 1992). It has been associated historically with cognitive changes secondary to atherosclerosis. However, it appears that the cerebral vasculature plays a relatively minor role in the changes typically observed in these patients. Although pathophysiology of the disorder is not clearly understood, the brains of patients at autopsy have been shown to contain numerous senile plaques, neurofibrillary tangles, and Hirano bodies. There is also marked degeneration of nerve cells. Although there is a slight increase in neuronal loss (about 5% per year greater than would be expected from aging effects alone), the dramatic atrophy sometimes observed on CT scans appears to be secondary to the shrinkage of neurons and loss of dendritic spines rather than to simple loss of neurons (Wolf, 1980). Neuronal shrinkage is most prominent in the association areas of the cortex, and there is relative sparing of the sensory and motor cortex in the early stages of the illness. The severity of symptoms will correlate directly with the mass of tissue lost, the density of senile plaques and neurofibrillary tangles, and the degree of ischemic softening present. Although this process is pathological in the case of Alzheimer's disease, by the tenth decade of life virtually every human brain is found to contain senile plaques and tangles.

Computerized tomography frequently fails to show brain pathology in the patient with early Alzheimer's disease, even in the case of a clearly demented patient, and *functional measures (such as performance on psychological tests) offer a better assessment of impairment than does tomography, and are consistently better predictors of remaining lifespan*. Positron emission tomography (PET) scanning holds considerable promise as a diagnostic tool for assessing patients with Alzheimer's disease (Freedland, Budinger, Brant-Zadowski, & Jagust, 1984); however, the technology is not widely available. The average lifespan from the time of diagnosis to death is slightly more than seven years, with considerable variation across patients (Strub & Black, 1988).

The etiology of Alzheimer's disease is not well understood. It appears that there is a genetic component to the disorder; 43% of monozygotic twins are concordant for the disorder, compared with 8 % of dizygotic twins (Lishman, 1978). Aluminum toxicity, choline deficiency, and virus exposure have all been investigated as causal agents.

A seminal study conducted at the Albert Einstein College of Medicine revealed the presence of a protein antigen in the brains of 28 Alzheimer's patients, which appears to be absent in normal brains (Wolozin, Pruchnicki, Dickson, & Davies, 1986). This work is exciting because it holds promise as a marker for the disease. The diagnosis of Alzheimer's is traditionally made by exclusion of other causes of dementia; the presence of a clear marker will greatly facilitate diagnosis and research, and, if the protein is found to be linked to a virus, our understanding of the disorder will be enhanced and new treatments will be developed.

Wells and Duncan (1980) have delineated three characteristic stages in the progression of dementia. In the early stage, there are multiple vague symptoms that are often diagnosed as functional. There are multiple somatic complaints that do not fit easily identifiable patterns. Complaints of weakness, insomnia, constipation, and dizziness are common, as are depression and irritability. There is apt to be confusion in response to very slight provocation (e.g., a change in appointment times), and this behavior is usually inconsistent with premorbid personality. The patient will frequently make excuses for poor performance ("I've never been very good at math"). *Memory deficits are especially common and will frequently be the chief complaint*: Patients find that they have to struggle to complete what used to be easy tasks, and they may make excessive use of notes, lists, and schedules. *It is rare for the medical/ neurological evaluation of the patient to be positive in the early phase of the illness; however, cognitive deficits will typically be apparent on neuropsychological screening.* Neuropsychological findings will prove most valuable when they are inconsistent with educational or vocational history.

It is important to appreciate that many patients become quite good at rationalizing their failures. Friends and coworkers may deliberately conspire to cover-up the mistakes and mishaps of the patient. One of the authors once saw a patient who was clearly demented but who continued to go to work each day; on questioning the patient acknowledged that he was "pretty much carried by my union brothers." Patients may also cope with their loss of cognitive skills by deferring to other family members during questioning and by claiming that the questions or the testing procedures being employed are foolish and a waste of time. *When neuropsychological screening does occur, motor skills are apt to be found to be intact and intellectual skills as measured by the Wechsler Adult Intelligence Scale–Revised (WAIS-R) are likely to be relatively well preserved in contrast to performance on more sensitive screening tests such as Trails B and the Category Test.*

In the middle phase of the dementing process the patient's difficulties with orientation, memory, judgment, and problem solving become apparent, even with a rudimentary MSE. Mood is apt to be flat or labile, and there is typically diminished concern for appearance and personal hygiene. There are clear changes in personality and behavior. Primitive reflexes may emerge, and the psychologist may find it valuable to systematically test for abnormal reflexes. In the patient with primitive reflexes, a grasp reflex can be elicited simply by lightly stroking the patient's hand. A rooting reflex may be elicited by stroking the corners of the patient's mouth to see if he turns his lips toward the stimulus. This response is normal in infants. A snout reflex will be demonstrated by the puckering of the patient's lips in response to gentle tapping on the lower lip with a pencil. Finally, a palmomental reflex will be observed in some demented patients. This occurs when the patient retracts one side of his mouth and chin in response to gentle stroking of his palm.

The psychologist will have little to contribute to assessment of the patient in the late phase of dementia. This phase is characterized by profound apathy and personality disturbance, with impairment of all mental, motor and sensory abilities. By this stage the patient is frequently bedfast and will typically be incontinent for both urine and feces. Brain mass and weight are reduced, and there is often a global aphasia.

In the early stages of Alzheimer's disease, it is common for both the electroencephalogram (EEG) and the computed tomographic (CT) scan to remain normal. With progression of the disease, the EEG will typically display mild diffuse slowing, whereas in many cases the CT scan will come to show ventricular enlargement and widening of the cortical sulci. There are decreases in both cerebral oxygen uptake and cerebral blood flow.

The WAIS-R is not especially sensitive to early dementias. If it is given, the psychologist will typically find that performance scores are lower than verbal scores. The Wechsler Memory Scale is apt to be more sensitive to the cognitive changes seen in dementia than is the WAIS-R, and one would expect to find memory quotients lower than full-scale IQ scores. There is frequently considerable subtest scatter across the WAIS-R scales. Screening measures such as Halstead's Category Test and Part B of the Trail Making Test are likely to indicate clear cognitive impairment (Strub & Black, 1981). Mild dysnomia is frequently evident in patients with an early dementia, and tests of verbal fluency (such as the Controlled Word Association Test) may prove to be especially sensitive (Cummings, 1985).

Table 1.1 lists many disorders that can potentially be treated if identified. It is especially tragic when a patient with a reversible illness (normal pressure hydrocephalus, for example) is misdiagnosed as having Alzheimer's disease and is sent to a nursing home when a correct diagnosis and appropriate treatment could have alleviated the symptoms that were present.

Pick's disease is a currently untreatable degenerative dementia that must ultimately be differentiated from Alzheimer's disease on the basis of histological findings. It is one-fifth as common as Alzheimer's and tends to affect the cerebral hemispheres differentially, producing more damage in the frontal and anterior temporal lobes (unlike Alzheimer's, which is characterized by more parietofrontal and hippocampal involvement). Because of the strong frontal involvement, patients with Pick's disease lose social graces early in the progression of the disease, and disinhibition is common. Many of these patients will develop echolalia. The Pick's patient is somewhat less likely to develop a seizure disorder but is more likely than the Alzheimer's patient to develop signs of the Kluver-Bucy syndrome (orality, hyperphagia, hypersexuality, placidity, and sensory agnosia). To some extent, attempts at differential diagnosis are an empty intellectual exercise, because diagnosis does not lead to specific treatment. The experimental treatments that have been proposed (e.g., choline and vasodilators) have not yielded significant clinical improvement for either disease.

Repeated vascular occlusions or small hemorrhages can produce a multiinfarct dementia that is almost always accompanied by a history of hypertension. The neuropsychological picture is characterized by rapid onset with a stepwise pattern of deterioration. The neurological and behavioral signs associated with multiinfarct dementias are more dramatic than those found with an Alzheimer's patient, but memory is likely to be better preserved in the multiinfarct patient. In addition, the patient with vascular disease is more likely to develop a pseudobulbar state (e.g., prolonged and exaggerated laughing or crying). In contrast to Alzheimer's, the patient with a multiinfarct dementia is slightly more likely to be male.

A number of other degenerative diseases can produce the syndrome of dementia. We can only mention a few of the more important ones here; however, more detailed descriptions are available in any standard neurology textbook.

Although James Parkinson believed there was no cognitive decline with the disease that today bears his name, more recent evidence suggests he was wrong; although it is mild, there is an unquestionable dementia present in at least half of patients with Parkinson's disease (Lechtenberg, 1982). Specific neuropsychological deficits can be demonstrated in over 90% of patients with Parkinson's disease when appropriate tests are used (Cummings, 1985). Deficits tend to be in the areas of orientation, constructional abilities, and memory, with social behavior and language relatively spared.

The most salient symptoms of Parkinson's disease are bradykinesia (slowness of movement), rigidity, and a resting tremor. In addition, the clinician should look for a masklike and expressionless face, diminished blinking, poor posture and balance, a shuffling gait, and the presence of involuntary "pill-rolling" movements. Micrographia is also frequently present. These patients are often clinically depressed, and may be taking antidepressant medication along with L-dopa. Psychiatric symptoms commonly develop in response to the necessary medication regimen.

Parkinson's disease results from loss of the capacity to produce dopamine in the basal ganglia. Parkinson's disease can be idiopathic, postencephalitic, or drug induced. It typically affects people over the age of 50. Men develop Parkinson's disease slightly more often than women.

Dementia is also a characteristic features of Huntington's chorea, another basal ganglia disorder, which causes selective destruction in the caudate and putamen. The disease is an autosomal-dominant disorder, with onset of symptoms typically in the age range of 45 to 55 years.

Unfortunately, many victims of Huntington's disease have already had children by the time their disease is diagnosed. Fifty percent of these children will also develop the disorder. *A positive family history is the single best predictor of Huntington's chorea; however, it is frequently denied by patients or the cause of the parent's death may be unknown.*

The movement disorder that accompanies Huntington's disease involves both chorea (brief, nonrepetitive jerks of the fingers, extremities, face, and trunk) and athetosis. Athetosis refers to the inability to sustain a particular group of muscles in one position, because of interruption by slow, purposeless movements. In Huntington's disease, flexion of the wrist with extended fingers is especially common. *The combination of athetosis and chorea of all four limbs is a cardinal feature of Huntington's chorea.* However, in the early stages of the disorder, the clinician may miss subtle signs, which the patient frequently disguises by making the movement appear voluntary (e.g., brushing his hair back). We recommend asking the patient simply to sit still with his arms outstretched and his eyes shut; if it is present, the movement disorder should be apparent in this condition. Other motor problems can include facial grimacing, swaying, and lurching of gait. The movement disturbances frequently are exacerbated by stress and disappear with sleep.

Cognitive and personality changes frequently precede the development of movement disorders. Unlike many other dementias, the patient with Huntington's disease is acutely aware of his failing mental powers. This may contribute to the very high suicide rate that is present in these patients. In rare cases, onset of symptoms may begin in childhood or adolescence; early onset generally predicts a more rapid and severe deterioration. Death usually occurs within 15 years after the onset of the disease.

Multiple sclerosis (MS) should be mentioned along with the other dementing illnesses we have discussed because it is important in the differential diagnosis of a variety of neurological disorders and because in rare cases, dementia may be the initial presenting symptom. MS is a chronic degenerative disease, which typically destroys myelin in the white matter of the brain and spinal cord. The disorder strikes women slightly more often than men, and it usually first presents between the ages of 20 and 40. The disorder is quite rare before age 10 or after age 50. It occurs with greater frequency in individuals who reside in colder climates, and several studies suggest that people who migrate in childhood from colder climates carry an increased risk, even though the disease may not become apparent until 20 years or more after their migration.

MS is characterized by an unpredictable course with irregular exacerbations and remissions. Exacerbations may be triggered by stress, fatigue, temperature change, poor health, or menstruation. Primary presenting symptoms include weakness or numbness in one of the legs; a variety of visual disturbances, including diplopia; loss of visual acuity and visual field defects; brainstem defects such as vertigo and vomiting; gait disturbance; and disorders of micturition. Patients also sometimes display inappropriate affect, including euphoria and eutonia (a general feeling of pervasive physical well-being). Scanning speech (slowed speech with pauses between each syllable), along with tremor and nystagmus, are sometimes found (these three signs are referred to as Charcot's triad); however, *it is critical for the clinician to appreciate that there are no truly typical presenting signs and symptoms in multiple sclerosis; it must be considered as part of the differential diagnosis with every patient who presents with a confusing clinical picture*. Ultimately, the diagnosis has to be made on the basis of history, although some patients may have CSF abnormalities, pale optic discs, and clear abnormalities on visual, auditory, or somatosensory evoked potentials. Magnetic resonance imaging (MRI) also shows great promise as a tool for diagnosing multiple sclerosis. Neuropsychological impairment typically involves loss of memory for recent events and impairment of conceptual thinking (Golden et al., 1983).

Wilson's disease, also known as hepatolenticular degeneration, is an autosomal recessive genetic disorder of copper metabolism. It appears primarily in childhood and early adulthood. Although it can occur at any age, its first appearance is rare after age 40. It presents in many ways like Huntington's disease. However, *Wilson's disease is a classic masquerader: at least 20 % of cases will initially present solely with psychiatric symptoms such as anxiety, depression, mania, or paranoid thinking*. These patients are often initially treated by a psychiatrist or psychologist.

The suicide rate for patients with Wilson's disease is quite high. It is critical that all psychologists be alert to the possibility of the disorder, because early treatment can reverse much of the damage that may have occurred. Treatment involves use of a chelating agent, such as penicillamine, to lower serum copper levels and increase urinary copper excretion. Prognosis is good with early identification. Without treatment there is continuing loss of neurons in both the cortex and basal ganglia and increasing dystonia and dysarthria. Additional clinical signs of the disorder include the presence of a Kayser-Fleischer ring (a brown-green ring around the cornea that is pathognomonic for the disease), increased pigmentation of the anterior aspects of the lower legs, and blue-green lines running transversely across the fingernails.

Human Immunodeficiency Virus Dementia

It is sobering to realize that the first edition of this book did not require a section on AIDS-related dementia, AIDS dementia complex, or what is more accurately known as human immunodeficiency virus (HIV) dementia (or HIV organic mental disorder in the *Diagnostic and Statistic Manual* [DSM]-*IV*). Since publication of the first edition, AIDS and HIV infection have become even more serious public health problems, and researchers and clinicians have learned that HIV infection can result in a subcortical dementia.

Early researchers dismissed the behavioral changes they observed in HIV positive patients as sequelae of the emotional response to the disease, but recent studies have demonstrated that neurological complications occur in about 40% of patients with AIDS, and in 10% of these patients the neurological manifestations will constitute the first clinical signs of disease (Pajeau & Roman, 1992). In one study at The Johns Hopkins University, one patient in four presented with evidence of an AIDS dementia complex before any other clinical symptom was present (Dal Canto, 1989). Ho et al. (1989) reported that 80% to 90% of the brains of AIDS patients they examined demonstrated neuropathological abnormalities.

About 10% of cases of AIDS occur in people 50 years of age and older (Scharnhorst, 1992), and it is important that HIV dementia be considered in the differential diagnosis of older patients suspected of having a dementing illness. This discrimination is often not easily made, and there is perhaps no other area in which there is so much overlap between psychiatric conditions (e.g., acute stress reactions, adjustment disorders, reactive psychoses, and depression) and neurological disease.

Sarbin (1987) has referred to AIDS as "the new great imitator," and it must be considered along with multiple sclerosis, Parkinson's disease, and Alzheimer's disease when patients present with nonspecific neuropsychological findings. At the very least, the clinician should search for risk factors for AIDS. If they are present, serological testing should be recommended (Maj, 1990).

Patients with HIV dementias present with cognitive, motor, and behavioral symptoms. The cognitive signs of HIV dementia include memory disturbance, lack of ability to concentrate, and confusion. The onset of these symptoms is insidious. Motor symptoms include loss of balance, clumsiness, and weakness in the lower extremities. Behavioral symptoms include apathy, blunted affect, social withdrawal, and loss of libido. Depression is a frequent complaint, and the psychomotor slowing observed in these patients resembles that found in clinical depression; however, when depression accompanies HIV dementia, it is resistant to treatment with medication.

On neurological examination, the patient with an HIV dementia will often exhibit gait ataxia and hyperreflexia. *Dysdiadochokinesis* (difficulty executing rapid alternating movements) is common. Other neurological symptoms such as tremors, primitive reflexes, or myoclonus may be present. Evaluation with computerized tomography or MRI (the more sensitive measure) often shows cortical atrophy, dilated ventricles, and white matter disease.

Neuropsychological evaluation of patients with HIV dementia remains the most sensitive measure for identifying the early and subtle changes associated with this disorder, and it provides far more sensitive data than that available from standardized mental status examinations (Pajeau & Roman, 1992). Although the difficulties documented by neuropsychological testing will be a function of the severity and stage of the disorder, it is common to find that patients with HIV dementia have difficulty with tasks requiring complex sequencing, fine rapid motor movement, processing speed, and visual scanning (Redmond & Wilson, 1990).

Butters et al. (1990) have proposed an extended (7 to 9 hours) and a brief (1 to 2 hours) neuropsychological battery for assessing the cognitive changes that occur in HIV seropositive, asymptomatic individuals. The recommended tests are listed in Table 1.3. Almost all of these tests are discussed in detail in subsequent chapters in *Screening for Brain Impairment*.

Although HIV dementias result in cortical changes (e.g., cerebral atrophy), they are generally regarded, along with Huntington's and Parkin-

TABLE 1.3   Domains of the NIMH Core Neuropsychological Battery

A. Indication of Premorbid Intelligence
   1. Vocabulary (WAIS-R)[a]
   2. National Adult Reading Test (NART)
B. Attention
   1. Digit Span (WMS-R)
   2. Visual Span (WMS-R)[a]
C. Speed of Processing
   1. Sternberg Search Task
   2. Simple and Choice Reaction Times
   3. Paced Auditory Serial Addition Test (PASAT)[a]
D. Memory
   1. California Verbal Learning Test (CVLT)[a]
   2. Working Memory Test
   3. Modified Visual Reproduction Test (WMS)
E. Abstraction
   1. Category Test
   2. Trails Making Test, Parts A and B
F. Language
   1. Boston Naming Test
   2. Letter and Category Fluency Test
G. Visuospatial
   1. Embedded Figures Test
   2. Money's Standardized Road-Map Test of Direction Sense
   3. Digit Symbol Substitution
H. Construction Abilities
   1. Block Design Test
   2. Tactual Performance Test
I. Motor Abilities
   1. Grooved Pegboard
   2. Finger Tapping Test
   3. Grip Strength
J. Psychiatric Assessment
   1. Diagnostic Interview Schedule (DIS)
   2. Hamilton Depression Scale[a]
   3. State-Trait Anxiety Scale[a]
   4. Mini-Mental State Examination[a]

[a]Instruments included in the abbreviated version of the NIMH neuropsychological battery.

Source: Butters, N., et al. (1990). Assessment of AIDS-related cognitive changes: Recommendations of the NIMH Workgroup on neuropsychological assessment approaches. *Journal of Clinical and Experimental Neuropsychology, 12*, 963. Reprinted by permission.

son's disease, as *subcortical dementias* because of the salience of the white matter changes that occur with the disease (Navia, Jordan, & Price, 1986). In general, cortical dementias result in specific deficits such as aphasia, agnosia, amnesia, and acalculia. Subcortical dementias spare language but result in dysarthria, abnormal posture and gait, bradykinesia, and movement disorders such as chorea, rigidity, ataxia, and tremor (Kaemingk & Kaszniak, 1989). The distinguishing features of subcortical and cortical dementias are presented in Table 1.4.

HEAD TRAUMA

Head trauma is the leading cause of brain injury for children and young adults, and it is estimated that 7 million head injuries and half a million related hospital admissions occur annually in the United States (Bond, 1986). It is an area of critical importance in neuropsychology because *detailed psychometric assessment will frequently reveal deficits in the head injured patient when all other neurodiagnostic tests are negative.* The psychologist must be sensitive to the medical sequelae that can result from trauma and must appreciate the physics of head trauma as well as have a basic understanding of the structure of the brain and skull to approach the head-injured patient with any real understanding of the nature of the injury. In addition, the general clinician must be sensitive to possible untoward developments, such as cerebrospinal rhinorrhea (leakage of CSF from the nose secondary to a traumatic fracture of the cribriform plate), which may signal the need for immediate medical referral because CSF leakage provides an easy route for subsequent brain infection.

Traumatic head injuries are traditionally classified as concussions, contusions, or open-head injuries. The concussion occurs when the brain is jarred. Strub and Black (1988, p. 316) define a concussion as "an acute impairment of cerebral function secondary to an impact injury to the head in which the following are usually, but not invariably, present: amnesia, loss of consciousness, and complete recovery." The amnesia can be either retrograde (for events prior to the moment of injury) or anterograde (for events that occurred subsequent to the injury); neither type of amnesia necessarily predicts permanent brain injury. However, with *repeated* concussions, permanent damage is likely to occur. This chronic condition is referred to as traumatic encephalopathy. It is also knowm as dementia pugilistica or punch-drunk syndrome because of its frequent occurrence in boxers. The syndrome is clearly evi-

TABLE 1.4   Distinguishing Features of Subcortical and Cortical Dementias

Characteristic	Subcortical dementia	Cortical dementia	Recommended tests
Language	No aphasia (anomia, impercipience if severe)	Aphasia early	FAS test Boston Naming test WAIS-R vocabulary
Memory	Impaired recall (retrieval) > recognition (encoding)	Recall and recognition impaired	Wechsler memory scale: Symbol Digit, Paired Associate learninq (Brandt)
Attention & immediate recall			WAIS-R-digit span
Visuospatial skills	Impaired	Impaired	Picture arrangement, object assembly and block design; WAIS subtests
Calculation	Preserved until late	Involved early	MiniMental Status
Frontal systems abilities (executive function)	Disproportionately affected	Degree of impairment consistent with other involvement	Wisconsin Card Sorting Task; Odd Man Out test; Picture Absurdities
Speed of cognitive processing	Slowed early	Normal until late in disease	Trail making A and B; Paced Auditory Serial Addition Test (PASAT)
Personality	Apathetic, inert	Unconcerned	MMPI
Mood	Depressed	Euthymic	Beck and Hamilton Depression Scales
Speech	Dysarthric	Articulate until late	Verbal fluency Rosen, 1980
Posture	Bowed or extended	Upright	
Coordination	Impaired	Normal until late	
Motor speed and control	Slowed	Normal	Finger-tap; grooved pegboard
Adventitious movements	Chorea, tremor tics, dystonia	Absent (Alzheimer's dementia—some myoclonus)	
Abstraction			Category test (Halstead Battery)

Source: Cummings, J.L. (1990). *Subcortical dementia* (p. 7). New York: Oxford University Press. Reprinted with permission.

dent in many aging boxers and includes dysarthric speech, slowness of thought, emotional lability, mild paranoia, and difficulty with impulse control. A good illustration of dementia pugilistica is available in the Martin Scorsese film *Raging Bull*.

A more common result of even a single concussion is the controversial postconcussion syndrome, characterized by problems with memory, impaired concentration, headaches, intellectual and physical fatigue, anxiety, dizziness, and increased sensitivity to noise. Impotence and irritability are also frequently noted following concussions.

Contusions are more serious traumatic injuries in which the brain is actually bruised, typically from its impact with the skull. The contusion can result either from direct bleeding at the site of impact or from the tearing of adjacent blood vessels connecting the brain and meninges. The behavioral effects of the contusion last longer than those of the concussion, and the neuropsychological findings tend to be more focal. Basal frontotemporal contusions occur most frequently. The contusion can produce a *coup* injury at the point of impact; this is most common when a moving object (e.g., a blackjack) hits a stationary head. *Contrecoup* injuries occur when a moving head hit a stationary object (e.g., when a head hits a steering wheel during a motor vehicle accident); these injuries are characterized by damage to tissue opposite the site of impact and occur with most cases of posterior head injuries that produce marked frontal and anterior temporal lobe damage in those areas where the brain rebounds against the opposite end of the skull. In contrast, contrecoup injuries to the occipital lobes themselves are quite rare, probably because of the smooth contour of the occipital bones and the absence of bony projections on the inner side of the posterior skull (Reitan & Wolfson, 1985).

Open-head injuries and brain lacerations occur most often in wartime. They produce focal lesions, but the resulting edema and bleeding may result in diffuse damage with multiple behavioral deficits. Patients with open-head injuries typically make rapid progress, and the majority of those who survive their injuries return to work. A combination of frontotemporal injury and low premorbid IQ are the best predictors of an inability to continue working after an injury (Lezak, 1983). If the injury severs a major cerebral artery, pronounced deficits and eventual death are the most likely outcomes.

Many head-injury patients will be comatose for days or weeks after their injuries. The duration of coma has been shown to correlate well with mortality, psychosocial dependency, and intellectual impairment, especially in patients over the age of 30 (Strub & Black, 1988).

TABLE 1.5   The Glasgow Coma Scale

Eyes	Open	Spontaneously	4
		To verbal command	3
		To pain	2
	No response		1
Best motor	To verbal command	Obeys	6
response	To painful stimulus[a]	Localizes pain	5
		Flexion-withdrawal	4
		Flexion-abnormal (decorticate rigidity)	3
		Extension (decerebrate rigidity)	2
		No response	1
Best verbal		Oriented and converses	5
response[b]		Disoriented and converses	4
		Inappropriate words	3
		Incomprehensible sounds	2
		No response	1
Total			3–15

[a]Apply knuckle to sternum, observe arms.
[b]Arouse patient with painful stimulus if necessary.

Source: Teasdale, G., & Jennett, B. (1974). Assessment of coma and impaired consciousness: A practical scale. *Lancet, ii*, 81. Reprinted with permission.

The Glasgow Coma Scale (Table 1.5) provides a convenient and objective method for rating level of consciousness. The scale assesses three areas: eye opening, motor responding, and verbal responding. Each area is scored, and scores are summed; the summed scores can range from 3 to 15. A score of 15 indicates that the patient is alert and responsive; a score of 3 indicates a deep coma. Patients with scores of 7 and below are considered to be comatose. The Glasgow Coma Scale is discussed in greater detail in chapter 5.

The total duration of post traumatic amnesia is a more useful predictor of degree of injury and likelihood of recovery than either retrograde amnesia or the length of time a patient is comatose. It is also a significant predictor of the length of time before a patient can return to work.

Table 1.6 lists the conventional nomenclature for rating the severity of head injuries. Note that the duration of posttraumatic amnesia is measured from the time of the injury until the restoration of continuous

TABLE 1.6   Relationship between Posttraumatic Amnesia and Severity of Injury

PTA	Classification
< 1 hour	Mild
1–24 hours	Moderate
1–7 days	Severe
More than 7 days	Very severe

awareness; islets of memory do not qualify as evidence of restoration of memory functioning.

Most closed-head injuries produce deficits that implicate both hemispheres. Motor and sensory deficits tend to be less pronounced than those that accompany vascular disorders. However, traumatic vascular injuries such as epidural, subdural, subarachnoid, and intracerebral hemorrhages are frequent concomitants of both open- and closed-head injuries. Injuries to the frontal lobes are common, resulting in loss of inhibition and behavioral control and impaired ability in simultaneous processing and in processing complex stimuli. Memory skills are frequently impaired. *Traditional measures of global intellectual ability are frequently insensitive to the effects of head injuries because the handicap that results from a head injury is not one of intelligence but rather one of attention, memory, and a broad range of information-processing skills* (Bond, 1986). Head-injured patients deserve to be assessed with measures at least as sensitive as those we discuss later in this book. If at all possible, they should receive a comprehensive neuropsychological workup.

SEIZURE DISORDERS

Epilepsy is not a disease in its own right, but rather a symptom complex characteristic of a variety of disorders that alter brain function. It can be defined as the recurrent paroxysmal uncontrolled discharge of cerebral neurons in such a way as to interfere with normal activity. Seizure activity is most often the consequence of head trauma: seizures develop in about 5% of closed-head injuries and in more than 30% of head injuries where the dura has been penetrated (Lishman, 1978). A variety of other disorders can insult neural tissue, including birth trauma, infectious disorders such as meningitis, toxins such as mercury, vascular changes, metabolic or nutritional disturbances such as electrolyte and water imbalance or vitamin deficiency, neoplasms, and degenerative diseases such as multiple sclerosis. The disorder is termed *idiopathic epilepsy* when no discernible cause is present for the seizures which occur.

The incidence of epilepsy is approximately 1/200 in the general population, with the occurrence decidedly higher in males. There are approximately two and a half million epileptics in the United States today, 20% of whom are not adequately controlled by medication.

Seventy-five percent of seizure disorders begin before the age of 20; 30% begin by the age of 4. Less than 2% of seizure disorders have their onset after the age of 50 (Trauner, 1982). *Onset of seizures in a patient after the age of 35 without clear causation must always lead to the presumptive diagnosis of a brain lesion, and these patients require immediate neurological evaluation.*

A number of environmental stimuli may precipitate seizures in the susceptible individual. These include hyperventilation, sleep deprivation, sensory stimuli, trauma, hormonal changes, fever, emotional stress, and drugs (Pincus & Tucker, 1985).

Classification of seizure activity has always been somewhat arbitrary, imprecise, and sometimes confusing. However, the International Classification of Epileptic Seizures has been widely accepted. This classification schema is reproduced in Table 1.7.

Partial seizures are so named because seizure activity begins locally and only part of the brain is involved. Partial seizures with elementary symptoms involve focal motor or sensory symptoms (such as a twitching finger), which may escalate along one side of the body (a "Jacksonian march") but which by definition never come to involve the entire brain and body. The motor disturbance usually begins distally and moves in a proximal direction, and the patient remains conscious throughout the event.

Partial seizures with complex symptoms are of particular interest to the psychologist. These seizures have traditionally been called psychomotor seizures, or sometimes temporal lobe seizures (somewhat incorrectly, because they can also originate in the inferior medial aspects of the frontal lobe). These are the most common form of seizure, and their first occurrence is typically around the age of puberty. Although the origin is focal, these lesions result in symptoms that are complex and varied. There is a prodromal period that may be characterized by feelings of impending disaster. During the ictal event itself, the patient experiences an altered state of awareness and may hallucinate. Feelings of *déjà vu* (in which new experiences seem familiar) and *jamais vu* (in which familiar settings or situations seem unusual and unreal) are com-

TABLE 1.7 Outline of the International Classification of Epilepsy

I. Partial seizures (seizures beginning locally)
    A. With elementary symptomatology (generally without impairment of consciousness)
        1. With motor symptoms
        2. With special sensory or somatosensory symptoms
        3. With autonomic symptoms
        4. Compound forms
    B. With complex symptomatology (generally with some impairment of consciousness)
        1. With impairment of consciousness only
        2. With cognitive symptomatology
        3. With affective symptomatology
        4. With psydiosensory symptomatology
        5. With psychomotor symptomatology (automatisms)
        6. Compound forms
    C. Partial seizures, secondarily generalized
II. Generalized seizures (bilaterally symmetrical without known local onset with loss of consciousness)
    A. Absence
    B. Tonic/clonic
    C. Tonic
    D. Clonic
    E. Bilateral epileptic myoclonus
    F. Atonic
    G. Akinetic
    H. Infantile spasms
    I. Myoclonic
III. Unilateral seizures
IV. Unclassified seizures

mon. Oral or facial automatisms such as blinking, smacking, and chewing are often present. While seizing, the patient will move about and may interact with other people in his environment; however, the *person having partial complex seizures will not engage in structured, purposeful, and sequential activity.* (Jack Ruby's lawyers argued that he was experiencing a psychomotor seizure when he shot Lee Harvey Oswald. However, it is unlikely that a seizure patient would be able to carry out the complex chain of events required to complete an assassination successfully. In general, the incidence of violent behavior in psychomotor seizures is quite low.) After a seizure the patient is typically confused and depressed, and there is a total amnesia for the events of the ictal period.

Hallucinations are common in partial complex seizures, especially with seizure foci in the posterior part of the temporal lobe. Visual hallucinations are the most common (18%), followed by auditory (16%), olfactory (12%), and gustatory (3%) hallucinations. Rage reactions occur in about 2% of cases, while the sensation of déjà vu occurs in 14% of seizures. Visual hallucinations originating in the temporal lobe tend to be complex and detailed, while those that originate in the occipital area are simpler and appear as colored lines, stars, and circles in the contralateral visual field. *When auditory hallucinations occur with partial complex seizures they are usually unformed and the contents are rarely bizarre, threatening, or condemning* (Kilpatrick & Hall, 1980).

There has been a great deal of interest in the "temporal lobe personality," which is believed to be associated with partial complex seizures. Patients with complex partial seizures often exhibit emotional lability, sudden outbursts of anger, circumstantiality, and decreased frustration tolerance. They are also noted to be hyperreligious, hyposexual, viscous, and hypergraphic. Hyposexuality results from loss of interest rather than from loss of ability. These patients also become quite serious about even minor matters and develop a fascination with details and minutia. Flor-Henry (1976) maintained that patients with right-sided foci were likely to be emotionally labile and eventually develop affective symptoms, while patients with left-sided lesions experience paranoid or grandiose delusions and eventually develop a schizophreniform psychosis.

Generalized seizures are bilaterally symmetrical and involve both hemispheres of the brain. Their origin is deep in the brain, and these seizures result in loss of consciousness. In *absence* (petit mal) seizures there is a brief (5- to 15-second) loss of consciousness without loss of muscle tone. The seizure is accompanied by a vacant stare and occasional eye blinking. The EEG almost always shows 3/second wave and pike discharges during the ictal event. The disorder occurs almost exclusively in young children, who may have multiple episodes each day. The diagnosis should be questioned if the phenomenon occurs fewer than five times per day (Lishman, 1978). The disorder is *not* associated with diminished intelligence, and the condition almost always clears after puberty.

Generalized tonic-clonic seizures (grand mal seizures) involve a sudden loss of consciousness with tonic rigidity followed by clonic jerking. The ictal event lasts for one to two minutes and may involve loss of consciousness, tongue biting, and urinary and fecal incontinence. Following the seizure there is a period of postictal confusion accompanied by headache and fatigue, along with a total amnesia for the ictal event.

Contrary to popular lore, nothing should be inserted in the mouth of the patient during the seizure episode; instead, the head should be protected and emotional support should be provided when the seizure ends.

Although the EEG will almost always be abnormal during an actual ictal event, the simple waking EEG will be normal in at least 50% of bonafide seizure patients. Greater accuracy occurs when sleep deprivation, photic stimulation, or hyperventilation studies are used. A left hemisphere EEG focus predicts diminished verbal IQ (relative to performance IQ scores), whereas the reverse is true with patients with a right hemisphere focus (lower performance IQ relative to verbal abilities). In general, the severity of neuropsychological impairment correlates well with longer duration and earlier onset of seizures. Neuropsychological impairment also correlates with seizure frequency, and tonic-clonic seizures are associated with a greater degree of neuropsychological deficits than complex partial seizures (Reitan & Wolfson, 1985).

2

Psychiatric Disorders with Neurological Implications

The distinction between neurological and psychiatric disorders is a false dichotomy, and the clinician must be alert for organic correlates and causes in every patient seen. However, for the sake of tradition and convenience, we follow the practice of separating neurological and psychiatric disorders and in this chapter briefly discuss the neuropsychological relevance of a variety of disorders traditionally viewed as functional. These clearly include schizophrenia and affective illness and, to a lesser extent, alcoholism. Each disorder will be discussed in turn.

SCHIZOPHRENIA

Most psychologists and other mental health workers have been trained to recognize schizophrenia. It is a common disorder with a worldwide incidence of at least 1%, and one cannot work for long in the mental health system without encountering a number of schizophrenic patients. However, perhaps because of its relative frequency, it is all too easy to overdiagnose schizophrenia; and we believe this occurs frequently in state hospitals and mental health clinics where there may be little time to perform a comprehensive diagnostic evaluation.

Schizophrenia is easier to recognize than define. Bleuler originally described the disorder in terms of four fundamental symptoms. He said the schizophrenic patient displayed defects in *association* and *affect* and was characterized by *ambivalence* and *autism*. Although conceptually neat and alluringly alliterative, there are a number of practical problems with Bleuler's criteria. Most importantly, Bleuler's symptoms lack precision. Schneider improved the situation somewhat by developing first-rank and second-rank criteria for the diagnosis of schizophrenia. Schneiderian first-rank symptoms include auditory hallucinations, delusional experiences, and distorted perceptions. Secondary symptoms include blocking, concrete thinking, and distorted ideas of reference. Pincus and Tucker (1985) listed six major criteria for the diagnosis of schizophrenia: (1) A thought disorder characterized by either hallucinations of delusions in the absence of some known cause, or some other form of conceptual disorganization, (2) early onset of symptoms, (3) absence of major affective symptoms, (4) absence of major neurological deficits, (5) a progressively deteriorating course or an intermittent course with remissions, and finally, (6) a history of schizophrenia in close relatives (which contributes to, but is not necessary for, the diagnosis). DSM-IV criteria include the presence of at least two of five specific signs (e.g., delusions, hallucinations, disorganized speech), deterioration from a previous higher level of functioning, and continuous signs of the illness for at least six months at some time in the patient's life. In addition, it is necessary to rule out schizoaffective and mood disorders, as well as substance disorders and general medical conditions that might account for the patient's symptoms. Psychological tests are specifically helpful in meeting this last criterion; however, *the diagnosis of schizophrenia is frequently made without consideration of the plethora of neurological disorders that can present with schizophrenia-like symptoms.* For example, unsuspected structural lesions are found in the brains of 5% to 10% of chronic psychiatric patients and meningiomas are found twice as often in psychiatric patients as in the general population (Lechtenberg, 1982). Many of the signs of schizophrenia (e.g., poverty of content, word salad, blunted affect) are found with specific neurological diseases and the effects of a lesion may mimic a schizophrenic process. We cannot emphasize strongly enough that patients suspected of being schizophrenic should receive neuropsychological screening to test for specific cortical deficits that may exist in addition to the more diffuse signs of schizophrenia. If specific neuropsychological deficits exist, medical referral is warranted.

Favorable prognostic signs in schizophrenia include sudden onset of the disorder, the presence of conspicuous precipitating factors, the pres-

ence of anxiety or affective symptoms, a family history of affective illness, a history of good social adjustment, marriage, employment, and
cooperation by the patient. Significant negative predictors include onset
of the disorder in childhood or puberty and a family history of
schizophrenia.

Although DSM-IV classifies schizophrenia into specific subtypes (disorganized, catatonic, paranoid, undifferentiated, and residual types), we
find it more useful simply to classify patients as being process or reactive schizophrenics. This dichotomy has been used by clinicians for
years in one form or another. Process schizophrenia is characterized by
gradual onset of illness, social isolation and withdrawal, and poor prognosis. Impaired performance on neuropsychological tests is almost always present. CT or MRI scans often reveal structural brain deficits, and
neurological soft signs are common. There is frequently a poor response
to neuroleptics. In contrast, reactive schizophrenia is characterized by
rapid onset and a better prognosis. Neuropsychological deficits are less
likely to be present, and specific neurological anomalies are rare. There
are fewer soft neurological signs on examination, and there is typically a
better response to medication. Reactive schizophrenics are characterized
by positive symptoms (delusions, hallucinations, and thought disorder),
while process schizophrenics are found to have primarily negative
symptoms (flat affect, little motivation, poverty of thought and speech).
Crow (1982) characterizes these as Type I (reactive) or Type II (process)
syndromes. *Although specific neurological deficits may be found in either group, evidence of brain impairment is far more likely to be
found in those patients with primarily negative symptoms.*

Neuropsychological assessment of psychiatric patients, particularly pro-
cess/chronic schizophrenics, has almost always yielded a high number of
what have traditionally been assumed to be "false-positive" diagnoses, since
these patients perform in a manner similar to patients with demonstrable
brain pathology (tumors, dementias, strokes, etc.). This finding, along with
the increased incidence of neurological soft signs (e.g., EEG abnormalities)
led some investigators to hypothesize that a sizable number of schizophrenics
did in fact have specific brain impairment. Recent technological advances,
such as computerized tomography, magnetic resonance imaging, and positron emission tomography, have supported this hypothesis. Compared with
normal controls, schizophrenics have larger cerebral ventricles, increased
sulcal widths, increased width of the interhemispheric fissure, cerebellar atrophy, and a reversal of typical patterns of asymmetry (i.e., wider left frontal
and right occipital lobes relative to normal controls). They also show decreased tissue density in the left hemisphere. These differences do not corre-

late with age, length of hospitalization, or medication use. Patients who demonstrate the greatest structural deficits tend to perform most poorly on neuropsychological tests and frequently have a poor response to chemotherapy (Wedding, 1986). Converging evidence from imaging technology, dichotic listening tasks, tachistoscopic presentation studies, psychophysiological research, and regional blood flow studies suggests (1) the anterior and dorsolateral portions of the frontal lobes are dysfunctional in schizophrenics and (2) the left hemisphere is more affected by the disease process than the right hemisphere. These findings are reported in detail in Henn and Nasrallah (1982) and Nasrallah and Weinberger (1985). It increasingly appears that schizophrenia research has come full circle, and we are once again at the point of trying to understand the neurobiology of "*Dementia Praecox.*"

Findings such as these illustrate the futility of attempting to find neuropsychological measures to classify patients into two arbitrary groups: psychiatric (functional) or neurological (organic). The dichotomy is artificial, and substantial overlap exists between the two populations. It is often more useful to describe the nature of the thought disorder that occurs in the schizophrenic patient and to screen for signs of specific focal damage that may point to remediable disorders (e.g., shunting in the case of normal pressure hydrocephalus).

Schizophrenia-like episodes have been associated with trauma, neoplasms, encephalitis, degenerative disease, autoimmune diseases, vascular disorders, and cerebral anoxia. However, Pincus and Tucker (1985) point out that disorientation, memory deficits, confusion, and fluctuating states of consciousness are more commonly encountered with specific neurological disease than with schizophrenia. In addition, acute neurological disorders are typically characterized by (1) a good premorbid social history, (2) abrupt changes in personality, mood, or ability, (3) rapid fluctuations in mental status, and (4) a lack of response to either psychotherapeutic or pharmacological intervention efforts.

Complex partial seizures can sometimes mimic schizophrenia, especially when there is a left sided anterior temporal focus (Flor-Henry, 1976). However, the absence of precipitating events, the shorter duration of bizarre behavior, the presence of an aura, and postictal drowsiness should help identify the recurrent complex partial seizure disorder.

AFFECTIVE DISORDERS

Affective disorders are the most common psychiatric condition treated in America today; they are also the disorders most commonly misdiagnosed as dementias. Because of the ubiquitous nature of this problem, it is essential that the clinician be sensitive to the possibility that a major depression is present in the patient who presents with cognitive failure, because *affective illness frequently mimics primary degenerative dementia, especially in the elderly*. In addition, many medical conditions present with depression as a primary initial symptom: these examples include anemia, multiple sclerosis, Cushing's disease, thyroid and parathyroid disease, acromegaly, systemic lupus erythematosus, and ulcerative colitis (Hall, 1980). In addition heart disease and cancer can initially present with the symptoms of fatigue and depression.

The problem of diagnosis is complicated by the fact that while depression can mimic organic mental syndromes, it can also be a part of the presenting picture of true brain disease. This is common with the catastrophic reaction that sometimes accompanies left-hemisphere lesions.

Although some authorities minimize the effect of depression on neuropsychological test performance, we have found the differential diagnosis of dementia and depression one of our most challenging (and most common) referral questions. It is a situation in which *good performance is more helpful than poor performance: good performance can help rule out brain disease, while poor performance does little to rule in the diagnosis of organic mental disease.*

Although poor test performance is characteristic of the patient with a major affective illness, some general principles can help the clinician make a more positive diagnosis. For example, in the depressed patient it is common for complaints and concerns about failing memory to be worse than objective performance on memory examinations. *Poor performance on tests of immediate memory and retention only should alert the clinician to the possibility of depression.* In addition, the psychologist often finds that verbal tasks are more helpful than nonverbal tests, since depressed people typically perform quite poorly on those nonverbal tests that require motoric responding. This is especially true when the test is timed. (Construction tasks are a possible exception. Given sufficient time most depressed patients can adequately reproduce simple geometric forms, while the demented patient may have a great deal of difficulty). Across a variety of tests, depressed patients tend to display deficits suggestive of frontotemporal deficits, with the right hemisphere tests more impaired than the left.

The psychologist should be especially sensitive to the likelihood of pseudodementia when performance on a screening battery is inconsistent from test to test, especially when similar abilities are being assessed by two separate tests. "I don't know" responses and paucity of effort are common in depression, but, with encouragement the patient will often respond correctly. However, it may be difficult for the truly depressed patient to maintain a consistently acceptable level of energy and effort, especially on tests such as the Digit Symbol subtest from the WAIS-R. We have found it helpful to administer the Controlled Word Association Test (discussed later in this book) to patients we suspect of having pseudodementia. Not surprisingly, a content analysis frequently reveals the presence of numerous responses suggestive of hopelessness and helplessness. Patient affect also may be diagnostically important. Although facial immobility of the depressed patient will sometimes resemble that of the patient with Parkinson's disease, more commonly one finds depressed affect that may prove helpful in differential diagnosis. Any family history of affective illness or suicide, as well as any past personal history of mood swings or manic episodes, may be diagnostically important as well.

Other dimensions separate the demented patient from the patient with a pseudodementia. There is more commonly some precipitating event (e.g., retirement or the death of a spouse) in depression, and the depressed patient is less likely to try to hide mistakes or to make excuses for poor performance on psychological testing. A history of marked guilt (occurring *before* the development of impaired cognition) suggests depressive pseudodementia. Associated vegetative signs of depression (e.g., weight loss, early morning awakenings) can occur with organic mental syndromes but are more common with depression. Progressive deterioration of functioning on serial testing would be more likely to occur in the patient with true brain disease, and a simple "Spike Two" profile would be somewhat less likely on an MMPI taken by a patient with an organic illness. *A positive Dexamethasone Suppression Test (i.e., failure to suppress cortisol secretion in response to administration of dexamethasone) suggests endogenous depression but is not definitive in ruling out organic mental disease.*

There are other differences between the patient with true dementia and the patient with pseudodementia. With true dementia onset of symptoms is insidious, with a gradual course; with pseudodementias the onset is more acute and the course more rapid. The demented patient often finds that his or her symptoms are exacerbated in the evening (sundowning); the depressed patient is likely to complain that his or her problems are worse in the morning. Adamant refusal to cooperate with testing is more common in the demented patient, while the depressed individual is more likely to cooperate superficially but put forth little effort on the actual tests that are administered. Finally, in the early stages of a dementing illness, social skills are likely to be well preserved, while they will be clearly impaired in the patient with a pseudodementia.

ALCOHOLISM

The practicing psychologist will frequently see patients whose cognitive functions have been adversely affected by substance abuse. Alcohol is clearly the single most abused toxin in the United States today, and there are estimated to be 9 to 12 million problem drinkers in the United States alone (Horton & Wedding, 1984). It is critical that the clinician be sensitive to the effects of alcohol on brain function because *cognitive impairment and cerebral atrophy will appear long before significant liver damage or other overt medical signs of alcoholism*. Psychological screening for cerebral impairment and memory dysfunction may be especially important in these patients, because social and verbal skills are relatively preserved and the existence of brain dysfunction may not be readily apparent on medical examination or on a casual MSE.

Korsakoff's psychosis is the brain syndrome most clearly associated with chronic alcoholism. This disorder is characterized by impairment of recent memory that is markedly greater than other cognitive deficiencies. Remote memory is also impaired, but to a less striking degree. These memory deficits are actually secondary to nutritional inadequacy and result from shortages of thiamine in the diet of the alcoholic that contribute to degeneration of the cortical mantel and atrophy of the thalamus and mammillary bodies.

Patients with Korsakoff's disease present with flattened affect and typically have little insight. They are likely to deny both the severity of their alcohol abuse and the significance of their memory failure. Immediate memory as measured on tests such as Digit Span tends to be intact, and oftentimes relatively good performance is present on most subtests on the WAIS-R. However, there will typically be at least a 20-point discrepancy between full-scale IQ and the memory quotient as measured by the Wechsler Memory Scale–Revised. Marked deficits will be present on any sort of delayed memory task, and confabulation may be present. *However, contrary to popular clinical lore, confabulation is neither consistently present nor is it a requirement for the diagnosis* (Adams & Victor, 1977). The personality changes associated with Korsakoff's disease most often involve passivity and apathy.

While the diagnosis of Korsakoff's disease highlights the presence of memory impairment, the condition almost always accompanies

Wernicke's disease, a disorder characterized by the triad of mental confusion, gait ataxia, and ocular abnormalities. The patient with Wernicke's disease is characterized by a wide-based stance and a slow and uncertain gait. Ocular abnormalities include ophthalmoplegias (weakness or paralysis of conjugate gaze) and nystagmus. The confusional state tends to be global, with the specific impairment of memory alluded to above. Since these memory deficits are virtually always present, many authors refer to this condition as Wernicke-Korsakoff's syndrome.

Space limitations preclude a more detailed discussion of the full range of psychopathology likely to be encountered by the clinician. The varieties and vicissitudes of mental illness and brain disease are such that a primer of this sort can only highlight the most common problems that occur. However, whatever the problem, the history and the mental status examination always will be critical parts of the clinician's data base. These areas will be discussed in the following chapters.

3

Approaches to Neurological Assessment

A neurologist is a physician who specializes in disorders of the nervous system. Most of the patients seen by a neurologist have been referred by other health care professionals who have performed their own assessments. If a complete physical examination has not been performed, the neurologist will perform one prior to the neurological examination. For these reasons, the neurological evaluation is different from that which would be conducted by most other health care professionals. The neurological evaluation concentrates on an assessment of nervous system functions. Although in most neurological evaluations, all areas of nervous system function are likely to be screened, more in-depth assessments are reserved for those areas that have been identified as problematic either in the history or in the referral. Despite the heterogeneity of neurological evaluations, they are all likely to be organized around certain areas of nervous system functioning. The neurologist will generally test the functioning of the cranial nerves, the cerebellum, the motor system, the sensory system, the reflexes, and the cerebral functions. The following descriptions are cursory and are only intended to inform the general clinician of the procedures that are likely to occur after the patient is referred to a neurologist.

The neurologist uses tests in a somewhat different way from the psychologist who associates the word "test" with a set of procedures that have rigidly standardized administration and scoring procedures. In the psychological test, measurement results in a numerical score that is interpreted via reference to a set of normative data. For the neurologist, a test is a set of procedures that are more loosely standardized. There is more improvization occurring in a neurological examination than in a psychological test.

The information derived from a neurological test is usually dichotomous. For example, in testing the reflexes, a set of fairly standardized procedures may be used to elicit the reflex. The information derived is whether or not the reflex occurred following the eliciting stimulus. Sometimes this information is qualified by an indication of whether the reflex was normal, exaggerated, or minimal. However, in contrast to the psychological test, scoring the neurological test is by comparison with a set of informal, internal norms. The neurologist decides whether the reflex is normal by comparing it with other reflexes that she has seen.

THE NEUROLOGICAL EVALUATION

The outpatient neurological evaluation begins when the patient walks in the door. The inpatient evaluation begins when the physician walks in the hospital room. The neurologist will pay attention to numerous aspects of the patient's behavior throughout the evaluation. During the initial interview, the neurologist will note the hygiene, grooming, and general appearance of the patient. The neurologist will also note the ability of the patient to use language and use this information to formulate the later assessment of language functions.

Arousal

The neurologist will assess the level of arousal of the patient, sometimes using one of the methods discussed in the section on arousal in the chapter of this book dealing with the MSE and sometimes using a more informal method. If the patient appears to be unresponsive to verbal stimulation, the neurologist may evaluate the responsiveness of the patient to tactile stimulation including responsiveness to painful stimulation. The level of alertness is noted, and a subjective narrative of the level is usually stated in the report.

History

The next step in the neurological examination is usually to take a detailed history. Because the neurologist is especially interested in aspects of the history for which the general clinician may have only a passing interest, the neurological history is likely to go into more depth than is the history taken by the general clinician. The neurologist will also perform a MSE similar to the MSE described in this book. However, the MSE given by the neurologist is less likely to make use of psychological tests and is more likely to use informal procedures for the assessment of mental status. If there is a suspicion that the individual is exhibiting cognitive impairment, the neurologist may refer to a neuropsychologist for a more in-depth assessment of cognitive processes.

Movement and Posture

The neurologist will next examine the station and gait of the patient. Station, or posture, is evaluated when the patient walks into the room, while the patient is sitting during the interview, and while the patient is performing those tasks suggested by the neurologist. Consistent leaning to one side is noted as is the level of muscle tone in relaxed and active states. Sometimes the Romberg test is used. In this procedure, the patient is asked to stand with his feet side by side and touching each other. The ability of the patient to maintain an even posture and to remain erect without swaying is evaluated. If the individual being tested sways with eyes closed but can stand with minimal swaying with eyes open, the test is said to be positive. Sometimes the patient will also be asked to stand on one foot to evaluate the same processes. The patient may also be asked to walk in a straight line, first freely and then heel to toe. A more difficult task requires the patient to hop on one leg for a short period. In all of these procedures, the strength, accuracy, speed, coordination, symmetry, and completeness of movement are assessed.

Cranial Nerves

An essential component of the neurological evaluation is the examination of the cranial nerves. The cranial nerves are a set of 12 pairs of nerves that connect the CNS processors with the rest of the body. The olfactory cranial nerve (I) is evaluated by providing the patient with odiferous substances, separately to each nostril, and asking the patient to identify the substance. Substances used include soap, coffee, wintergreen, camphor, or tobacco. (Because damage to the first cranial nerve is rare, this portion of the evaluation of cranial nerves is sometimes omitted.)

The optic nerve (II) is examined by testing visual acuity and visual fields. These tests are informal and may be followed up by more extensive testing procedures if the clinician deems it to be necessary. The oculomotor nerve (III) is assessed by examining for ptosis, appropriate dilation in response to light, and both the standing gaze and the ability of the eyes to follow a visual stimulus as it moves across the field of vision. The trochlear nerve (IV) is also assessed by examining the ability of the patient to track a stimulus. If the patient is unable to look downward and laterally, then the trochlear nerve is most likely affected. If the patient is unable to look laterally in one eye, then the respective abducens nerve (IV) is suspected of pathology. These symptoms are usually associated with complaints of diplopia. During this part of the evaluation, the neurologist is also examining for the presence of nystagmus. Cranial nerves III, IV, and VI are usually tested together.

The trigeminal cranial nerve (V) has a variety of functions that are assessed. Sensation for touch, pinpricks, heat, and cold are evaluated on both sides of the face while the patient's eyes are closed. By touching the cornea of the patient with a cotton swab, the neurologist can assess the corneal reflex. The neurologist will also ask the patient to close his jaws tightly, and then the neurologist will palpate the patient's jaw muscles in this part of the neurological examination. Finally, the maxillary reflex is tested by tapping the middle of the patient's chin when the mouth is slightly open.

The facial nerve (VII) is tested by examining the ability of the patient to imitate movements such as wrinkling the forehead, frowning, and raising the eyebrows. The patient is asked to tightly close his eyebrows, and the neurologist will attempt to open the eyelids with his hand. The sense of taste, which is also associated with the VII cranial nerve, is assessed by placing salt and sugar on the anterior portion of the tongue.

The assessment of the acoustic nerve (VIII) has two major areas of evaluation that reflect its double set of functions. The tests of the vestibular functions of the VIII cranial nerve involve rotation and caloric tests requiring specialized equipment and complex procedures, and are therefore not usually included in the routine evaluation. The cochlear functions of the VIII cranial nerve are more amenable to clinical examination. The patient is asked to close one ear with a hand and the ability of the patient to detect the sound of a ticking watch at 3 to 4 feet is assessed. The sensitivity of the patient to vibrations from a tuning fork is assessed as the fork is held near each ear as well as when the fork is in contact with the mastoid and the vertex of the skull. In addition, audiometric testing is sometimes used.

The glossopharyngeal nerve (IX) is tested by touching the posterior wall of the pharynx with a tongue depressor, which should result in contraction of the pharyngeal muscle. The results of this part of the evaluation are interpreted with reference to the results of the assessment of the vagus because it is possible that the pharynx is innervated by the vagus in some patients. When this is true, the contraction of the pharyngeal muscles will be accompanied by a gag reflex.

The vagus nerve (X) is assessed by examining the palate, larynx, and pharynx. The patient is asked to perform simple verbalizations (the proverbial "Ah") while these muscle groups are examined. The patient is also asked to swallow.

The accessory nerve (XI) is assessed by having the patient turn her head against the neurologist's hand while the sternocleidomastoid muscle is palpated. The patient is also asked to shrug her shoulders while the trapezius is palpated.

The hypoglossal nerve (XII) is examined by asking the patient to stick out the tongue, to move the tongue in and out rapidly, and, finally, to wiggle it from side to side. Additionally, the patient is asked to roll the tongue upward and downward. Finally, the patient is asked to lick her lower lip.

These procedures are not a comprehensive assessment of all functions associated with the cranial nerves. Some of the functions, such as the vestibular functions associated with the acoustic nerve, require special equipment. Other functions such as the sensory functions associated with the vagus are too difficult to assess clinically. However, these procedures will provide the neurologist with an idea of the relative integrity of the cranial nerves. If the evaluation results in the identification of deficits or if functions are suspected of deficit, more rigorous evaluation may be performed.

Tests of Sensation

The sensory evaluation has been described as the most difficult and least reliable portion of the neurological assessment. This part of the evaluation starts by asking the patient about feelings of numbness, tingling, crawling sensations on the skin, coldness, or burning. The patient's sensitivity to tactile sensation is also evaluated. Light touches, hard touches, and pin pricks are used to determine whether the patient feels the stimulation. Patterns of sensory recognition versus absence of recognition are compared with the known distribution of sensory neurons in the dermatones. Sensitivity to vibration is also assessed. The patient's limbs will be moved passively, and the patient will be asked to state the direction of the movement. The blindfolded patient will be asked to identify the site of tactile sensation. Finally, two-point discrimination may be tested.

Tests of Strength and Tone

The motor system is assessed by examining muscle tone and strength. The neurologist will examine the muscle groups looking for fasciculation, atrophy, or tremors. The neurologist will also examine the patient for signs of abnormal tone, such as spasticity, rigidity, or flaccidity. The neurologist will also examine for signs of chorea, tics, tremor, or myoclonus, and will ask the patient to flex and extend her muscles both without resistance and when the neurologist provides resistance contrary to the movement.

Reflexes

Testing for certain reflexes is part of the evaluation of cranial nerves. However, some reflexes are not covered by the examination of cranial nerves and need to be examined separately. The reflexes are divided into deep and superficial reflexes. The deep reflexes are tested by tapping a certain area of the body while that part of the body is relaxed. The speed and the strength of the reflex are compared with reflexes seen by the neurologist in other individuals. The deep reflexes include (with their normal responses) the biceps (contraction of the biceps), the brachioradialis (flexion of the elbow and pronation of the forearm), the triceps (extension of the elbow), the patellar (extension of the knee), and the Achilles (plantar flexion of the foot).

The superficial reflexes are tested by stroking the skin with a pointed object. The superficial reflexes include (with their normal responses) the upper abdomen (umbilicus moves up and toward the area being stroked), the lower abdomen (the umbilicus moves down), the cremasteric (the scrotum elevates), the plantar (the toes flex), and the gluteal (the skin tenses at the site of the stroke).

There are still other tests for pathological reflexes. These tests are for reflexes that were appropriate at an earlier age of development but that should not be present in the healthy adult individual. These include the Babinski reflex in which the lateral aspect of the sole is stroked. The abnormal response is an extension or dorsiflexion of the big toe and fanning of the other toes. In the Chaddock reflex the lateral aspect of the foot below the lateral malleous is stroked. The abnormal response is an extension or dorsiflexion of the big toe with fanning of the other toes. The abnormal response for the Oppenheim and Gordon reflex is the same, although the stimulation changes. The stimulation for the Oppenheim reflex is stroking the anteromedial surface of the tibia. For the Gordon reflex, the stimulation is a firm squeeze of the calf muscles.

Following the completion of the neurological examination, the neurologist may order further tests and lab work to provide more information before establishing a firm diagnosis. However, the further work is usually only to determine a differential, the alternatives of which have been reached by use of the neurological examination.

NEURODIAGNOSTIC TECHNIQUES

If the neurologist suspects the presence of a neuropathological condition, she may order a more extensive workup of the client. Depending on the problem, several alternative procedures may be used. To acquaint the general clinician with some of these procedures, we will now give brief descriptions of the procedures and the circumstances under which they might be useful.

Electroencephalography

The EEG is a means of evaluating the electrical processes in the brain. There are several types of EEG available. The most common type involves the use of surface electrodes to record the electrical activity at several sites on the scalp. Another type involves nasopharyngeal leads to record the electrical activity. Nasopharyngeal leads are used to record electrical activity that has its origins in the basal aspect of the frontotemporal areas; however, they are rarely used because of the discomfort caused the patient. EEGs can be taken when the patient is awake or asleep. Because sleep deprivation tends to accentuate EEG abnormalities, the EEG is sometimes recorded under those conditions. The EEG can be useful in the diagnosis of seizures disorders, but many patients with seizure disorders may have normal EEGs. Large tumors or cerebrovascular lesions may result in focal signs in the EEG. The EEG can also be useful in the diagnosis of encephalitis, degenerative processes, and metabolic encephalopathy.

Average Evoked Potentials

The average evoked potential is a variation of the EEG. In the average evoked potential (AEP), the patient is given some form of stimulation, usually auditory, visual, or somatosensory. The EEG in response to the stimulation is recorded over several sites and averaged into a single wave. The AEP allows the neurologist to measure the time it takes to process the stimulation, therefore facilitating estimates of conduction time. The AEP is useful in the diagnosis of demyelinating diseases, but the utility of AEPs for other disorders is not as well established.

Brain Electrical Activity Mapping

Brain electrical activity mapping (BEAM) is a relatively new technique that is used to assess differential levels of activation in the brain during a given task. In this technique, 20 electrode leads are attached to the surface of the scalp similar to the procedures used for EEGs. However, with BEAM, the information from the leads is used to estimate the activity in adjacent brain areas that are not directly measured. This is accomplished using a regression procedure to predict activity in a nonmeasured area by using the values obtained at the three closest leads and the distance of the area from the leads. This information is computer analyzed, and the output is a three-color map of relative levels of activation in different areas of the brain. The BEAM procedure can be used in either a process EEG methodology or a discrete event evoked potential methodology. Although relatively new and somewhat experimental, BEAM has been reported to be useful in the identification of pure dyslexia (Duffy, 1981); dementia (Duffy, Albert, & McAnulty, 1984); and in epilepsy, cerebral infarctions, tumors, and learning disabilities (Duffy, 1982).

Skull Radiographs

Skull radiographs are often used to determine the presence of structural deficits in the head. Although in the past, skull radiographs have been used to diagnose degenerative disorders, tumors, inflammatory conditions, and even Cushing's disease (by documenting the thickening of vertebral endplates), they have been supplanted by the CT scan. However, skull radiographs are still useful in the evaluation of the acute effects of trauma.

CT Scan

The CT scan is actually a series of radiographs that are taken at different levels, or slices, of the brain. The results of each set of radiographs are fed into a computer that uses an algorithm to combine the different exposures into representations of the relative densities of structures in the brain. The CT is useful in the diagnosis of structural abnormalities such as tumors, cerebrovascular lesions, cerebral atrophy, and congenital anomalies. By first introducing a contrast material into the vascular system of the brain, the CT can be used to help differentiate between cerebral hemorrhage and edema. The use of contrast medium can also be helpful in determining the nature of a lesion (e.g., whether it is a glioblastoma or meningioma).

Regional Cerebral Blood Flow

Some neurological problems are metabolic rather than structural. In these cases, the neurologist may order a regional cerebral blood flow (rCBF). Although this procedure has shown promise in research settings, it has not been uniformly adapted in clinical settings. There are multiple methods, but the most common one is to have the client breathe oxygen that has been labeled with radioactive Xenon. To meet the metabolic requirements of brain activity, the oxygen travels to the areas in the brain that are being used. Multiple radioactivity monitors positioned on the client's scalp record the relative metabolic activity in these areas. In this way areas of decreased metabolic activity can be identified.

Positron Emission Tomography Scans

PET scans are a method by which an indication of the functional activity of regions of the brain is obtained. The PET has largely superseded the rCBF in many research settings. The PET scan technology involves having the subject ingest a small amount of radioactively labeled glucose and then engage in some cognitive activity. The brain areas with greater glucose use will show higher levels of the labeled glucose. Yet another use of the PET, although one with fewer clinical implications, is to label certain neurotransmitter ligands radioactively, thereby allowing identification of the sites in the brain where the transmitter is taken up by receptor sites.

Single-Photon Emission Computerized Tomography

Single-photon emission computerized tomography (SPECT) is gaining in popularity because it is much less expensive to use, and the technology is readily available in many hospitals. Here a chemical known as technetium-99m hexamethyl propylene amine oxime (HMPAO) is given intravenously to the subject. Uptake of the HMPAO is affected by rates of perfusion, allowing the clinician to evaluate differences in metabolic activity in regions of the brain. Both high and low levels of blood flow can then be documented; however, measurement is in only relative levels. Absolute levels of blood flow cannot be determined. Clinical applications are still developing.

Magnetic Resonance Imaging

The acronym MRI is the result of public concern over an earlier name for this procedure—namely, NMR, or nuclear magnetic resonance. Because that first name resulted in concern over "nuclear" activity in a hospital, the name was changed. MRI does not involve "nuclear" activity. It is based on the fact that nuclei spin, creating a magnetic field. Each type of nucleus has a particular spin with a signature magnetic field. When placed in a larger, stronger magnetic field, these nuclei will "hum" at an identifiable frequency. When a similar magnetic frequency is introduced, the nuclei absorb the energy and release this energy when the larger magnetic field is turned off. The strength of the signal sent out following turning off the larger magnetic field is proportional to the number of protons in a given area. By inducing various magnetic fields and turning them off, one can determine the relative amount of particular collections of protons. A computer can combine this information into "pictures" of the boundaries between different types of material that have different types of nuclei. The MRI procedures have been shown to be extremely useful in the diagnosis of multiple sclerosis, but other uses are experimental. Although at first it was hypothesized that the MRI would make the CT obsolete, at least one study has demonstrated the superiority of the CT in diagnosing acute subarachnoid or acute parenchymal hemorrhage (Snow, Zimmerman, Gandy, & Deck, 1986). In recent years, we have seen the advance of MRI applications and technology. For example, by comparing two serial MRI scans; one under resting conditions and one under conditions in which the subject is engaged in some cognitive activity, the examiner can determine relative blood flow and thereby provide a measure of functional activity in regions of the brain. Currently, the most frequent use of MRI is to determine structural anomalies or intracerebral bleeds.

Cerebral Angiography

Cerebral angiography is a radiological technique for visualizing the vascular system of the brain. In this technique a small amount of radiopaque dye is introduced into the blood stream via the artery that is in question. Following the injection of dye, a series of quick x-ray exposures are taken. Each successive exposure documents the progress of the dye through the artery. In this way occlusions and other vascular abnormalities can be detected. Cerebral angiography can be useful in the evaluation of possible arteriovenous malformations, aneurysms, vascular tumors, and occlusions. It is generally used when other diagnostic techniques have not been successful because of concerns about the amount of radiation to which the patient is exposed, because of the possible irritation from the contrast material, and because of the possibly painful nature of the procedure.

Lumbar Puncture

In some cases the neurologist may want to examine the composition of the cerebrospinal fluid. In this procedure, the patient is placed on his side, and his lower back is prepped. The patient is instructed to arch his back as he draws his knees toward his chin. A local anesthetic is given and a needle is inserted, usually in the fifth lumbar interspace. The needle is pushed into the patient until it punctures the dura. The pressure is monitored and then a sample of cerebrospinal fluid is drawn. The fluid can be tested for total protein, immunoglobulin, sugar content, the presence of bacilli, or the identification of malignant cells. This procedure has possible side effects of nausea, extreme headaches, dizziness, or neck pain. Therefore, it is used sparingly.

CONCLUSIONS

Although the neurologist and the neuropsychologist are both interested in central nervous system function, the evaluations used by the two types of professional vary. The neurologist is less likely to use standardized behavioral tests such as those used by psychologists. The neurologist is more likely to be interested in cranial nerve function than is the psychologist. However, there are many points of overlap in the structure of the two types of evaluations.

Like the neuropsychological evaluation, the neurological evaluation is a series of assessment techniques that are usually conducted in a hierarchical fashion. The first components of the evaluation involve a complete history and a clinical evaluation of cranial nerves and gross corticobehavioral functioning. If the neurologist suspects dysfunction but is unable to diagnose the exact condition, additional neurodiagnostic labwork may be ordered. The decision to pursue further evaluation is determined by the need for more information and the likelihood that the further tests will provide the necessary information.

4

The Neuropsychological History

A careful history is the most powerful weapon in the arsenal of every clinician, whether generalist or specialist. Brain-behavior relations are extremely complex and involve many different moderator variables, such as the age, level of premorbid functioning, and the amount of education. Without knowledge of values for these moderator variables, it is virtually impossible to interpret even specialized, sophisticated test results. The neuropsychological history is designed to obtain specific information regarding these moderator variables as well as to provide information related to risk factors such as exposure to neurotoxins.

For example a WAIS-R Full Scale (FS) IQ of 100 is considered average. However, obtaining a WAIS-R FSIQ of 100 tells us nothing about the possibility of acquired brain impairment unless we know whether this represents a change in the level of functioning for the individual under consideration. If a clerical worker presents with a FSIQ of 100, we might conclude that there have been no changes in general intellectual functioning. However, if a college political science professor presents with an FSIQ of 100, we would want to investigate the possibility that the score represents a decline in general intellectual functioning.

Research studies frequently attempt to diagnose individuals simply on the basis of single test scores. This type of research can be useful in the evaluation of the diagnostic accuracy of tests, but these tests were not designed to be used in that fashion. This sort of research, by its nature, attempts to isolate components of variables to examine them more carefully. Because test scores are the most easily quantifiable components of test performance, they are the most often used variables in the evaluation of the validity of tests. But the classification of individuals as brain-impaired simply on the basis of test scores is a simplistic and dangerous practice. The data from tests should always be integrated with information obtained through a clinical interview, information regarding the appearance of the person, and information regarding the qualitative aspects of performance.

Specialized fields have developed specialized interview techniques and questions. The general interview and the specialized interview are similar. They differ in the relative emphases placed on types of information and in the types of questions asked. In the specialized interview emphases are placed on investigating those variables that have been implicated in the relations between organic substrate and behavioral manifestations. Because of their training these specialists have become sensitized to certain issues.

APPEARANCE OF THE SUBJECT

The generalist clinician is already trained to pay close attention to the physical appearance of the subject. The specialist is further equipped with a set of definitions for terms that are used to describe abnormal aspects of appearance. There are multiple reasons why a subject may present an abnormal appearance, but when used in conjunction with the history and the test results, information regarding the appearance of the subject can be an aid in diagnosis or in the decision to refer to a specialist. In each case discussed here, it is not recommended that the generalist try to interpret the observations. Instead, observations of abnormalities should be used in the decision to refer, and such information should be passed along in the report to the specialist to whom a referral is made.

The evaluation of the client begins when he or she walks in the door. Is the client alone or accompanied? If alone, did the client possess enough memory skills to be able to remember the correct time and place of the appointment? Can the client ambulate under his or her own power? Does the client possess enough integrity of the visual-spatial system to find the location of the office accurately? Questioning the client can help determine whether the subject was able to navigate public transportation or the use of a private automobile to arrive at the evaluation.

The dress and hygiene of the subject can help the clinician to determine the level of recent attention to grooming. There are multiple reasons why an individual may show signs of personal neglect in physical appearance; depression and apathy are two common causes. Personal hygiene is also a reflection of cultural background. Although not all patients will share the clinician's sense of fashion or of usual, everyday hygiene, most people will share the value of appropriate grooming before coming in for an appointment with a health care professional.

Although rare, a readily observable pathognomic sign of organic impairment can be seen in the individual who dresses carefully on one side of the body but ignores the other side. This form of *unilateral neglect* will manifest itself in not properly buttoning or fastening clothes on one side of the body, or in men, in not shaving one side of the face. Somewhat more commonly, an individual may have poor hygiene over the whole body, but may not express awareness that something is amiss. This can be useful information, particularly if it can be ascertained that this is a recent development. Either of these observations may alert the clinician to the need for a more intensive MSE and ultimate referral to a specialist.

LANGUAGE ABNORMALITIES

When the patient enters the office, observations can be made regarding his capacity to initiate an interaction. Does the client spontaneously introduce himself? How are questions answered? Does the patient answer with single-syllable responses or is there amplification of the answer? If the patient answers with monosyllables, can they be encouraged to expand on his replies? What is the level of fluency? What is the apparent level of vocabulary? If there are questions regarding the vocabulary or fluency, a short standardized test such as the Vocabulary subtests of the WAIS-R or the Peabody Picture Vocabulary Test-Revised can be given supplemented by the Controlled Oral Word Association Test. *Dysfluency*, *dysarthria*, or other mispronunciation, and abnormal word usage are important signs of a possible aphasic disorder. If there are long latencies in answering questions, special focus on the Attention and the Language portions of the MSE may be warranted.

MOTOR ABNORMALITIES

Can the client enter the room with the effortless ease that we associate with the absence of impairment? What is the general quality of physical movement? Is the gait normal? Does the patient move readily in a straight line, or does she walk at an angle? Can the client walk around obstacles or does she bump into the doorjamb or into the furniture? Can the patient slow down and speed up her rate of movement in response to the requirements of navigation, or are changes in velocity jerky and abrupt? Are leg movements free and easy, or does walking appear to be an activity that requires much effort? Do the arms swing freely with the movements of the legs? Or is there either an excess arm movement or a tendency to keep the arms straight at the sides? Do the feet have a tendency to drop and point toward the ground when they are lifted in the walking movement, or are they kept relatively parallel to the ground as is normally the case? Abnormalities of motor activity in combination with cognitive deficits may point to the need for a referral to a specialist.

Observations of the quality of movement should continue throughout the evaluation. Because many of the procedures used in the MSE have motor components, many of these same questions should be asked when the client is required to write or draw. Additionally, certain types of movement have implications for the diagnosis of neurological and neuropsychological disorders. *Tremor* may be noticed either when the client is at rest or when the client is asked to perform some motor activity. The conditions under which tremors occur should be carefully noted. *Intentional tremors are more likely to be due to lesions near the motor strip, whereas at-rest tremors are more likely to be due to subcortical lesions.* In either case, referral to a specialist may be indicated.

The clinician should be alert for signs of a *tic* or other abnormal movements. Additionally, the clinician should note whether the tic occurs regardless of the situation, or if the tic's occurrence or rate is affected by requests to perform some activity or when an emotionally charged topic is discussed. *Choreiform* movements are rapid, repetitive stereotyped movements that involve larger groups of muscles than do tics. The whole lower portion of a leg or an arm may be involved in a choreiform movement. These movements lack purpose. The clinician must be observant because a client may have developed compensatory mechanisms to hide the choreiform activity. For example, one client developed a habit of scratching behind his neck to hide the fact that he had a choreiform movement that involved rapidly lifting his right arm behind his head. *Athetoid* movements are another motor abnormality. In athetoid movements there is an undulation of muscle groups. These may appear graceful, but they are involuntary and nonpurposeful just as are the general choreiform movements.

There is also a class of movement abnormalities that have as their root the word "tonia." In general, these refer to disturbances in the tonic level of muscle activity. *Hypertonia* refers to a state of sustained high muscle tension. *Hypotonia* is a state of low muscle tension. The extreme instance of this condition is *atonia*, which literally means a lack of muscle tone. Clients with this condition would be unable to come to an office for an outpatient appointment, but they might be seen in inpatient settings. The client may also show signs of *dystonia*, an involuntary motor activity that is slower and more sustained than choreiform activity. In addition, dystonia will usually contort the entire area of the body that contains the affected muscle group.

As well as abnormalities of tonic muscle condition, there may signs of abnormalities of the level of muscle activity. For example, a client may show signs of *akinesia*, which is a lowered level of muscle activity. Or there might be *akathisia*, which is motor restlessness as shown by pacing or continual movement associated with subjective reports of restlessness. For each of these conditions as well as for the conditions discussed previously, the reader is referred to chapter 1, which contains definitions of neurological and neuropsychological terms.

Abnormalities of symmetry can refer to either tonic muscle condition or to motor activity. However, these have different etiologies. For example, facial asymmetry may refer to asymmetry of the resting condition of the face, in which case, one side of the face may seem to droop, as in drooping eyelids (ptosis) or drooping at one corner of the mouth. Or there may be asymmetrical motor weakness, noticeable when the client is asked to perform a movement such as raising his eyebrows or smiling. Additionally, the clinician should be alert as to whether the asymmetry occurs during voluntary movements (such as during response to a command) or with involuntary movements (such as those associated with spontaneous expression of emotions). One should also assess whether the upper part of the face, the lower part of the face, or both areas are involved. *When the right side of the face exhibits weakness, the clinician should be alert for the existence of other symptoms that are associated with left frontal lesions such as right arm weakness and difficulty in producing fluent speech.* Especially if of recent origin, these signs indicate the need for referral to a specialist.

ESSENTIALS OF THE HISTORY

The overt purpose of the history is to obtain information that can be used in determining a diagnosis and in deciding whether to refer to a specialist. There are a series of questions that can be asked to obtain the necessary information. However, the observation of the client during the interview will also provide much useful information. In effect, the client tells us information with her verbal answers and with her associated behaviors. The earlier discussion in this chapter has focused on deriving information from the associated behaviors. We now concentrate on the types of verbal information that can be elicited from the client.

It is critical to first establish a form of rapport with the client. Clients are usually put off by the clinician who immediately starts asking questions. However, some balance needs to be struck because the clinician wants to communicate the message that she recognizes the situation as a professional exchange. The clinician can greet the client in a warm manner with a small amount of pleasant small talk but only until the client begins to feel at ease. It is helpful to begin the interview with straightforward, nonemotionally charged factual questions to further allow the client to adjust to the situation and to the clinician. In addition, we suggest that the clinician briefly address the issue of confidentiality. Although there is no need to concern the client unduly regarding the limits of confidentiality, it is preferable to describe the legal limits of confidentiality before the issue arises from the client's verbalizations. This is especially true for those clients who are court referred, or who may be involved in legal difficulties.

Identification of the Patient

The first few questions should relate to basic identifying information pertaining to the client. The clinician can ask for the client's name, age, nationality, and country of origin. One can neither assume nationality nor country of origin. In northern cities in the United States, accents may vary little across the Canadian-U.S. border. In the Southwest, U.S. citizens who grew up in bilingual households may exhibit Hispanic accents. Knowledge of the nationality of the client and the client's parents can help in interpreting data regarding the use or pronunciation of verbal material. If the country of origin is different from that of the current nationality, the clinician should determine how long the client has been in the country. The language that was used in the household of origin should also be determined. This should be done for all clients who report recent familial migrations to this country. In our experience it is not unusual to find clients from large cities whose families spoke Polish or Italian at the dinner table, especially if the household included the extended family and not just the nuclear family. All of these factors may affect a patient's performance on neuropsychological screening measures. Foreign origin or familial bilingualism reduce the diagnostic importance of poor performance on tests of language skills.

Current Complaints

Next the clinician should inquire as to the history of the current disorder. It is important to pay attention to not only what the client says but the way the information is presented. Does the client recognize the problem, or did he or she come into the clinic because of complaints from others in the environment? What are the symptoms? The clinician should probe for related symptoms. Clients may withhold information not out of a desire to mislead, but because he or she is unaware of the import of "trivial" symptoms (e.g., "trivial thirst"). Recent increases in thirst and in frequency of urination may indicate the onset of diabetes in patients who have initially come in with complaints of irritability, fatigue, or attention difficulties. Referral to a medical specialist is essential here.

For all symptoms, the clinician should inquire as to when the symptoms first occurred, whether the quality or severity of the symptoms have changed over time, and the effect of these symptoms on the everyday functioning of the client. Do others complain of the problem more often than the client does? How was the problem first noticed?

The clinician should also try to ascertain the extent to which the current level of symptoms represents a change. If a change has occurred, the clinician should ask whether the changes have been slow and gradual, or abrupt. This can be important information in determining the differential diagnosis. *If the changes have been abrupt and no traumatic event such as a blow to the head can be documented, then the hypothesis of a cerebral vascular accident should be considered.* Referral to a medical specialist is indicated. Similar to the information provided by abrupt changes, the quality of slow changes can provide information for the differential diagnosis.

Slow, gradual changes may reflect the presence of a dementing process such as Alzheimer's disease. Slow, stepwise changes that consist of a series of abrupt, but minor changes across different functions may reflect the presence of multi-infarct dementia. In multi-infarct dementia, the subject may first show an abrupt change in the ability to perform mental calculations and then a week later there might appear an impairment in short-term memory, and still later an impairment in a discrete area of language skills. A history of this type is common in the patient experiencing a series of small strokes in diverse areas of the brain.

A history of a series of discrete impairments that are temporary in nature may be the result of TIAs. *A person experiencing TIAs is at high risk for future strokes and should be referred to a neurologist immediately.* Prophylactic treatment in the form of diuretics will often reduce the danger from either multi-infarct dementia or TIAs. People suspected of having Alzheimer's disease should also be referred to a neuropsychologist or neurologist for further evaluation, but the element of time urgency is not as important as in the cases of TIAs and multi-infarct dementia.

Obtaining a history of the present complaints also involves investigating the environmental and behavioral concomitants of the client's complaints. Because we are biological as well as psychological beings, there are probably no complaints that will not have elements of both. However, the relative importance of these two variables will change from disorder to disorder and from case to case. The clinician should determine the antecedents and consequences of the occurrence of the complaint because symptoms may arise from varied causes. For that reason, it is critical that the clinician inquire as to whether the client is involved in litigation or had legal problems of any type as this may influence the appearance of symptoms.

In one case with which we are familiar, a client's complaints of memory impairment occurred 3 days after his notification that the compensation board had turned down his request for benefits based on a claim of black lung disease. The notification included the information that the board did not consider the client's degree of claimed impairment severe enough to warrant compensation. Whether the client was deliberately trying to mislead the clinician or did not mention his memory problem previously because he did not think it relevant to his application for benefits is immaterial. The fact remains that the memory complaints were linked to the environmental event of the notice from the disability board, and any evaluation would have been incomplete without this information.

In another case it was determined that a client's complaints of distractibility and short-term memory impairment were usually preceded by arguments with her teenage daughter who was dating a person whom the parents did not like and who was allowing her school performance to slide. Subsequent evaluations indicated that the client's problems were secondary to anxiety and stress.

Family History

The next area of information that should be investigated is the family history. The client should be asked about family history for psychiatric disorders because many psychiatric disorders like schizophrenia and major affective disorders have genetic components. The presence of family members with these disorders will help clarify the diagnosis of the subject. In a like manner, there are genetic components to several neurologic disorders. The report of family members who were diagnosed with Alzheimer's disease, hypertension, Huntington's chorea, or other related disorders should sensitize the clinician to the possibility that these disorders might be present in the client. The clinician should also inquire as to whether family members died early, or if there were family members who were mentally retarded or learning disabled. Not all clients will be able to recall this information. Therefore, it is a good idea to suggest that the client check out the information with other family members. In most families there is a "historian," usually a parent or grandparent, who can remember details about which the client may have no memory or no knowledge. One can suggest to the client that such a person be contacted to obtain a more complete history. Some clients may be sensitive about family history especially as it pertains to psychiatric disorders and suicide. The clinician should exercise tact and good judgment in questioning for this information.

Prenatal History

A history of prenatal events is a vital part of the history of the individual with suspected cerebral dysfunction. Unfortunately, it is routinely neglected by many clinicians. Fetal exposure to a wide range of toxins or infectious diseases can have severe effects on cognitive functioning later in life. The clinician should inquire as to whether the mother worked while pregnant and where this work was performed. Was the mother exposed to solvents, insecticides, or dyes? What was the mother's use of drugs during pregnancy? This applies to both prescription and recreational drugs. The case of thalidomide is only one example, albeit an extreme one, of the consequences of some drugs. The fetal alcohol syndrome is another example of how maternal drug use can affect later cognitive functioning. Prenatal maternal exposure to infectious diseases such as German measles can also affect the cognitive development of clients.

Complications in pregnancy can affect the cognitive development of the client. The client may not be an accurate historian for questions of this sort and should be encouraged to obtain the information from another source. Birth complications should also be addressed. Was the gestational age normal, premature, or late? Were there complications in the use of an anesthetic during birth? What was the weight at delivery? Was the use of forceps required?

Early History

Information about early development may have been transmitted to the client in the form of family stories, but these should always be verified whenever possible. The clinician can ask for permission to talk with a family member to corroborate information obtained from the client. The ages at which developmental milestones such as sitting up straight, walking, and talking were reached are important information. The clinician will also want to know about early posture and gait of the developing client. Whether or not the client experienced febrile convulsions should be determined. The presence of early developmental abnormalities may mean that there is a neurological substrate to the client's current complaints. This is not to say that all clients with early developmental abnormalities or delays will not have psychological disorders, only that the presence of developmental abnormalities tips the scale in the direction of deciding on a referral to a neuropsychologist or neurologist.

Personal development should be investigated. Did the client experience school phobias? Was the client able to form friendships while a child? What was the quality of these relationships? In general, the degree and type of social behavior is useful information in conducting this type of evaluation. It can help provide an estimate of whether the current complaints are recent or long-standing. For example, if a client reports that he had many childhood friends and was involved in intramural sports and other extracurricular activities, but currently lives alone and rarely goes out to socialize, we would hypothesize a change in social functioning.

An accurate academic history is necessary to interpret information from testing and other sources. It is not sufficient to inquire as to the highest grade completed. There are multiple reasons why a client may have terminated school early. Especially for older clients from a rural background, quitting school to help support the family by taking a job would not necessarily reflect limited intellectual capacity. Again, especially in rural states, compulsory education is a recent legal development. Clients may have grown up in an environment in which education was not valued and may have quit school because their peer reference group was doing the same thing.

Conversely, in recent times, we have witnessed the unfortunate phenomenon of social passing in school. Despite an inability or unwillingness to do the work necessary, the contemporary urban client may have been passed on to the next grade and may even have obtained a diploma. In all of the preceding cases, information about the grades earned by the client and the type of classes taken should be obtained. This information can be verified, with the permission of the client, by contacting the school involved or by contacting the person who was responsible for supervising the client during that time.

Occupational History

An occupational history is an extremely important aspect of this sort of evaluation. The occupation can give two types of information: an estimate of intellectual functioning and an estimate of social-behavioral functioning. These must be considered rough estimates as many people are underemployed, that is, they may be employed at a position that requires less than their maximum level of skills. However, the type of job held can be used as a lower limit estimate of intellectual functioning. For example, an individual who holds a job as a college professor of romance languages would be assumed to have a minimum level of intelligence and language skills. Complaints by this sort of person about problems with mental control, word-finding difficulties, and paraphasias represent serious impairment in ability.

Different jobs require different amounts of interaction with others. For example, a person with a job as a receptionist can be expected to possess a certain level of social skills. For such a client to come in complaining of irritability and impatience with people denotes change in the social functioning of the person. Other jobs, such as that of night watchman, require little interaction with others, and these clients cannot be expected to exhibit much in the way of social skills. Many night watchmen and other solitary workers may have more than adequate social skills, but this fact cannot be as readily assumed as it can in more people-oriented jobs.

Certain jobs may also expose workers to conditions that put them at risk for different disorders. The clinician should check to see if the client's job required working in a foreign country where exposure to infectious diseases might have occurred. A history of encephalitis or meningitis may account for later cognitive complaints. Other domestic jobs may involve exposure to chemicals that can have cognitive and behavioral consequences. Workers who are employed in factories that manufacture insecticides, fungicides, batteries, glass products, or solvents may come in with complaints of irritability, insomnia, loss of memory, impaired concentration, muscle weakness, or other problems. We know little about neurotoxins and their role in the development of neurological disorders. However, clients who come in with any of these complaints and who report that they work in environments where putative neurotoxins are manufactured or used should be referred to a neurologist or neuropsychologist for further evaluation.

Although we know little about the effects of most industrial chemicals on CNS functioning, there are a few chemicals for which we do possess some knowledge. The most infamous of these is mercury. The history of observed neurotoxic effects of exposure to mercury in the workplace dates to the Victorian period of Charles Dickens and Lewis Carroll. At that time mercury was used to fix the soft felt used in the manufacture of hats. Many of the workers in these plants developed psychological and behavioral problems including emotional lability, irritability, and illogical behavior patterns. This was how the phrase "mad as a hatter" originated.

Today we know that there are different effects for exposure to organic mercury and inorganic mercury. Exposure to inorganic mercury may result in complaints of anxiety, an unreasonable phobia for social gatherings, and disruptions in emotional functioning. Exposure to organic mercury, such as in the form of methyl mercury, may result in complaints of restlessness and in observations of slowed mental operations. Large, single doses can be fatal as in the incidence of fatalities seen in Japan in the early 1960s (Minimata disease) or in Iran in the 1970s when many people who ate bread made from grain treated with a methyl mercury compound died. However, even small levels of exposure over several years can result in the development of symptoms eventuating in referral to a mental health professional.

Other substances such as lead, arsenic, carbon disulfide, and manganese (Feldman, Ricks, & Baker, 1980) can also cause psychological and neurological symptoms. The clinician who suspects exposure to neurotoxins as an etiological agent should inquire as to gradual changes in appetite, sexual functioning, sleep patterns, memory, and emotional behavior. There are many possible symptoms including anorexia, incoordination, ataxia, hypertension, and perceptual disorders (O'Donoghue, 1985) and many different causes for any of these symptoms. However, if these symptoms can be reasonably associated with exposure to neurotoxins, a referral to a specialist who can arrange for a complete medical workup is indicated.

Sexual History

The next area to be addressed in the history is that of sexual functioning. In our culture sexual behavior is considered to be private, and many clients may demonstrate a reluctance to discuss such matters. Therefore it is a good idea to inquire about sexual functioning late in the interview, after the clinician has had a chance to develop a rapport with the client. Asking these sort of questions early in the interview may unnecessarily frighten off a client from making a full disclosure of relevant information. The clinician would be well advised to maintain an objective, professional demeanor during these questions to reassure the client of the clinical nature of these inquiries. Some clients may encouraged to provide this type of information. However, the clinician should never make light of the client's reticence or probe too hard as this is likely to alienate the client.

These questions should assess past as well as present sexual behavior. For women, one should inquire about the age of menarche and whether there are any past or present irregularities in the menstrual cycle. Not all women are uniformly regular in their menstrual cycles. However, any changes in regularity should be noted. In addition, the clinician can ask about abortions and the conditions under which these might have occurred. For men, questions should include the age at which puberty was reached. These can involve the age at which the client's voice started to crack, or the age of the first nocturnal emission or the first orgasm by masturbation.

For both sexes, the clinician should ask about the first sexual interactive behavior and other historical aspects of sexual behavior. Taking information about current sexual behavior would be insufficient because it would not allow the clinician to determine if a change had occurred. The question of homosexual behavior should be broached with sensitivity because of the values placed on this behavior by our culture. The presence of a history of promiscuous behavior, whether heterosexual or homosexual, can alert the clinician to the possibility of sexually transmitted diseases, many of which have CNS effects if not treated. In recent years the cognitive effects of AIDS have become more well known.

Changes in sexual behavior can have important implications for the current diagnosis. Decreases in sexual performance may be related to infectious diseases or exposure to neurotoxins. Decreases in sexual desire may be related to affective disorders. Impotence in men is commonly related to psychological problems, however it is wise to first rule out a physiological etiology.

Increases in sexual behavior may reflect either a neurological or a psychological etiology. Hypersexuality, reports of lowered need for sleep, incidences of spending sprees, and periods of extreme elation are often associated with manic-type bipolar affective disorder. Frontal lobe injuries such as those sustained in closed-head injuries may result in inappropriate sexual behavior associated with impulsivity. Changes in sexual behavior are also associated with subcortical tumors. The presence of changes in sexual behavior is not always associated with neurological disorders. However, information about sexual behavior is so important in establishing the correct diagnosis that the clinician who sidesteps the issue because of his own squeamishness is doing the client a disservice.

Medical History

A medical history is a necessary step in the initial evaluation of a client. This investigation should include long-term as well as recent history. Many childhood illnesses have CNS effects that are not present in adults. An example of this is German measles, which can lower intellectual functioning in children. The clinician should inquire about the occurrence of diseases such as meningitis, encephalitis, and epilepsy. The clinician should also inquire as to whether the client suffers from migraines or other headaches. Headaches may signal the presence of a vascular disorder or a tumor, especially if seen in conjunction with cognitive or emotional changes. There are many possible etiologies for headaches, but a medical evaluation is needed to provide the diagnosis.

Any form of surgery, but especially neurosurgery, should be completely documented. The clinician needs to know whether a general anesthetic was used and if there were any complications of the surgery, such as respiratory arrest or subsequent infections. In cases of respiratory arrest, there may be later problems with memory or attention, and those sections of the MSE should be emphasized. Any report of a closed-head injury should be amplified with information regarding whether hospitalization was required, whether there was a loss of consciousness, the duration of such a loss, and whether the subject exhibited post-traumatic amnesia. The duration of the post-traumatic amnesia should also be documented. Finally, the clinician needs to determine whether any behavioral patterns were changed following the injury and the duration of these changes. Subjects with closed-head injury often exhibit increased irritability and temper as well as decreased levels of patience.

It is evident that the client will be a poor historian, particularly in the case of closed-head injury. A person can rarely observe her own posttraumatic amnesia or loss of consciousness. Changes in behavioral patterns may also not be evident to the client. Once again, the clinician needs to contact someone in the patient's environment who was witness to the events or who is able to comment on changes observed in the client. We cannot emphasize enough the importance of corroborating information with a secondary informant in this or in other matters such as the determination of developmental milestones.

A psychiatric history should be taken from all clients. For most general clinicians, this portion of the history will not differ from the history that is usually taken. The first questions involve whether the person has experienced any problems in the past, the nature of these problems, and whether the person sought professional help for these problems. The clinician would be wise to remember that depression is most often first seen and treated by a general practitioner or family doctor and that many people refer their psychological problems to a member of the clergy for assistance. The type of treatment applied and whether the client felt the treatment was successful is important information. Unsuccessful counseling treatments for complaints of depressed affect may indicate an organic basis to the complaints. There is a big difference between the disorder that was successfully treated by pastoral counseling and the disorder that required long-term hospitalization. If the client has experienced problems in the past, the similarity of these problems to the current complaints should be elucidated.

A history of suicide attempts should always be investigated, and the presence of past or present suicidal ideation or suicide attempts should be documented. If there have been past attempts, the lethality of these attempts should be determined as well as the occurrence of hospitalization following the attempts. Not all suicidal reports need to be a cause of immediately hospitalizing the client, but all reports of suicidal ideation should be carefully evaluated. Furthermore, suicide attempts accompanied by hypoxia put a person at risk for the development of memory, attention, or abstraction deficits that should be examined in the MSE.

The use and abuse of drugs also needs to be investigated. In our culture the values placed on drug use may induce the client to underreport her incidence of drug use, just as the laws of our society may incline the patient to deny drug use. Drugs, including alcohol, have powerful CNS effects. The clinician needs to impress on the client the need for a completely accurate account of drug and alcohol use. Even at that, it is probably safe to assume that the levels of use reported by the client are an underestimation. If the abuse has not been long-term, some of the neuropsychological complaints such as impaired short-term memory and decreased attention and concentration may subside if abstinence is maintained for a period of six months. Unfortunately, most clients do not see a clinician until the effects of their substance abuse have become more widespread and in some cases permanent.

Determination of premorbid personality and behavior patterns is another area that requires corroborating information from a source in the client's environment. Some clients will be able to describe accurately changes that have occurred since the onset of the problem. However, it is more likely that clients will underestimate the degree of change or will deny that any change has occurred. In its most extreme form, this is a symptom known as *anosagnosis*, literally the inability to know one's impairment. Family members are good sources for this type of information because they have usually seen the client in many different situations across many developmental stages. Consistent changes are more readily noticed by them than by acquaintances. As mentioned earlier, changes in temper, impulsivity, or patience can follow neurological insult to the brain. The other extreme is also possible; clients may become more apathetic and withdrawn following a closed-head injury.

Human social interaction is a complex set of operations that require subtle perceptual mechanisms and higher order judgmental processes. If a person experiences a neuropsychological impairment in any of the cortical-behavioral skills required, he or she may withdraw from situations that require social interaction because of the confusion and embarrassment that these situations cause.

Forensic information also needs to be gathered in the history. Again, this type of information is sensitive and should be corroborated. The clinician should inquire for both present and past legal difficulties. A long history of legal scrapes may indicate long-standing adjustment difficulties. A current increase in legal problems may indicate recent neuropsychological impairment. For example, impulsivity subsequent to frontal lobe injury may result in an increase in "spur-of-the-moment" ill-planned illegal activity.

A woman who was referred to one of our labs was brought in by her adult children because she had had five minor traffic accidents in a period of 6 months. Testing revealed that despite the fact that she was able to conceal most symptoms from her children, she was suffering from a degenerative dementia. As another example, a farmer who developed a temporal lobe tumor started exhibiting irrational behavior. He took out a large loan, ostensibly to update his farm equipment and was unable to account for the money at the end of 4 months, ultimately defaulting on the loan.

Current Situation

Current litigation should be determined. The potential award of large sums of money can be a powerful contingency in shaping the motivation of a client. In these cases, every effort should be made to obtain the cooperation of the client in obtaining factual information and optimal test performance. Similarly, the threat of a jail sentence can influence the behavior of a client, making this sort of information invaluable to the clinician. Few clients are neuropsychologically sophisticated enough to malinger in a consistent and neurologically coherent fashion across a variety of tests assessing cortical behavior skills. However, the determination of malingering on neuropsychological tests is a decision best left to the specialist.

Finally, the current living situation of the client should be evaluated. Recent changes in living situation such as being asked to move out of a spouse's residence can reflect behavioral difficulties. Conversely, changes in the living situation of organically impaired individuals can result in an exacerbation of symptoms. This is most clearly seen in the case of Alzheimer's disease patients who become confused and irritable when even small changes in daily routine occur.

CONCLUSIONS

As discussed earlier in this chapter, the history can be a potent instrument in the evaluation of neuropsychological disorders. However, its power increases with the level of knowledge and skill of the clinician. This chapter can be used as an outline for taking a history, but the use of this outline does not guarantee success. With practice and experience the clinician will become more adept at using the history as a means of conducting a complete evaluation. But it is also recommended that the clinician consult neurological texts such as those by Pincus and Tucker (1985) or Adams and Victor (1981) and neuropsychological texts such as those by Golden (1978), Heilman and Valenstein (1985), or Grant and Adams (1986) to become acquainted with the clinical presentations and associated histories of various CNS system disorders.

5

The Mental Status Examination

The MSE can be a powerful tool in the repertoire of clinicians. The utility of the MSE can be seen in its adoption by several different disciplines. There are many different forms of the MSE that have been developed for use in areas such as neuropsychology, neurology, clinical psychology, psychiatry, and general medicine. Forms of the MSE sometimes also vary by particular institutions. The MSE that will be presented here is not unique. It borrows from formats used at the University of Nebraska, West Virginia University, and Marshall University.

The goal of a MSE is to obtain information that can be used in an initial formulation of the client's problems. Different forms of the MSE reflect the types of information that the different disciplines use in clinical practice. For example, the MSE used by neurologists may include testing the reflexes and cranial nerves of the patient. We do not recommend that clinicians use procedures with which they may be unfamiliar. The procedures presented here are ones that can be used by most individuals who have graduate training in clinical psychology.

The amount of information derived from a MSE and the utility of that information in arriving at a diagnosis are partially determined by the skill level of the clinician conducting the MSE. Conducting the MSE smoothly and quickly is a behavioral skill that can only be achieved via practice. However, the level of interpretation depends on the amount of formal training and supervised clinical experience of the clinician. We intend this MSE to be used as an initial screen in the decision to refer to a specialist. No clinician can ethically exceed his expertise by attempting to interpret beyond his level of training and experience.

This MSE is not intended to replace a comprehensive neuropsychological or neurological evaluation. If signs of organic involvement are present or if the results of the evaluation are questionable, the client should be referred to a professional specialist (neuropsychologist or neurologist) for a more complete evaluation.

When seeing a client for the first time, a complete history should be taken, especially if the client is self-referred. For most clients the MSE will take between ½ hour and 45 minutes. However, the length of the MSE will vary with the degree of the clinician's suspicion regarding the existence of organic impairment. Any areas that provide evidence for the presence of impairment should be followed up. This is not to say that areas that are not suspected can be safely ignored. Clients may come in with one complaint, and on evaluation, may manifest other, different impairments. Clients, like the rest of us humans, are not always the most objective judges of their conditions. Alternatively, clients may not feel comfortable relating all of the details of their problems. All areas, therefore, should be sampled, but in-depth evaluations may be required only in a portion of the areas sampled.

There are several classes of clients who can be considered a priori candidates for the extended MSE. These include clients with documented CNS lesions. The lesions can result from tumors, trauma (closed-head injuries or penetrating wounds as the result of automobile accidents, sporting accidents, barroom brawls, etc.), or CVAs (strokes). Another group of clients who should receive the MSE includes those with suspected CNS lesions. Although there may be no medical documentation of these clients' problems, they may complain of dizziness, seizure activity, headaches, or they may report a history of untreated head trauma. Some of these clients may report a history of metabolic medical disorders, such as meningitis or poorly controlled diabetes.

Clients with a report of sudden changes in emotional status, behavior, or in everyday aspects of cognitive functioning are also candidates for the MSE. For these clients, the information is more likely to originate from a source other than the client, such as a family member. There are many different reasons why sudden changes in behavior or emotional condition may occur. Obviously, many of these reasons are environmental, and a functional analysis can provide good information in determining the etiology of the changes. However, sudden changes can also be the result of unreported traumatic events. The client may not initially report a blow to the head especially if the blow did not result in unconsciousness, but careful questioning by the clinician can uncover this fact. Fast-growing tumors can lead to precipitous changes in behavior. When a tumor is the cause, these changes in behavior may be accompanied by discrete, focal impairment. Recent sensory impairment is often associated with organic involvement and any reports of sensory impairment should be followed with an extended MSE. Positive findings on the MSE indicate the need for referral.

Complaints of psychiatric symptoms should also be investigated with a MSE. There is a large body of evidence to suggest that some psychiatric disorders are associated with neuropsychological impairment. In fact, an important a question that is often faced by clinical neuropsychologists in psychiatric settings is the differential diagnosis of such individuals. Conversely, clients with neurological impairment will often present with psychiatric symptoms. There is not a strict dichotomy between neurological impairment and psychiatric impairment. Humans are complex phenomena whose various systems interact. It is therefore important not to think of a client as having one type of disorder, but rather to view the client as an individual with certain skills and deficits. Some individuals may have greater degrees of neurological impairment or of psychological and behavioral abnormality, but a pure case is rare.

BRIEF EVALUATIONS

Another class of patients for whom an extended MSE is recommended are those individuals for whom the clinician suspects cognitive impairment merely on the basis of clinical presentation. Of course this is subjective decision, the accuracy of which depends on the level of experience of the clinician with cognitively impaired individuals. In making these decisions, the clinician may elect to complete a briefer evaluation.

Folstein, Folstein, and McHugh (1975) have presented an instrument called the Mini-Mental State (MMS) for the rapid evaluation of cognitive functioning that can be used to make decisions regarding the administration of an extended MSE. The MMS can be given in about 10 minutes and is appropriate for use in patients with psychiatric or psychological disorders. The MMS provides a quick assessment of orientation to date and place (but not to time or person), of attention, delayed recall, and a few select aspects of receptive and expressive language functions. The MMS was reported to have a 24-hour test-retest reliability coefficient of 0.88 in a sample of 22 depressed patients, a 28-day test-retest reliability coefficient of 0.98 in a sample of 23 stable impaired subjects, and an interscorer reliability coefficient of 0.83 in a sample of 19 depressed subjects. Although the MMS appears to be able to identify cognitive impairment in neuropsychiatric patients and able to differentiate cognitively impaired subjects from nonimpaired subjects, it does not appear to be able to separate organically impaired subjects from schizophrenic subjects. However, a score of lower than 20 points is probably indicative of organic impairment, and patients obtaining such a score should be given an extended MSE or else referred for more intensive evaluations.

The MMS has been criticized for having a high rate of false negatives. In particular, the MMS may misclassify individuals with focal impairment or the beginning signs of dementia. However, the MMS remains the single most used short screening device, especially in medical populations. McNulty et al. (1993) report that only the attention items of the MMS did not differentiate their sample of a stroke and non-stroke subjects. In a different light, Starrat, Fields, and Cisewski (1992) reviewed the literature on the MMS and concluded that in clinical populations of older individuals, the MMS has reasonable relations with global measures of intellectual functioning, but that the relation of MMS scores to neuroimaging data and functional evaluations is more variable. Overall, the MMS is best thought of as a quick procedure where positive findings have more utility than negative findings.

Another short screening device that has generated recent interest is the Neurobehavioral Cognitive Status Examination (NCSE) (Northern California Neurobehavioral Group, 1988). This instrument provides a brief evaluation of level of consciousness, orientation, attention, language, constructional ability, memory, calculations, reasoning, and judgment. In the attention, language, calculations, reasoning, and judgment areas, the subject is given a single item. If the subject fails the item, it is followed by a few more items tapping the same skill area. Although the NCSE appears to be relatively sensitive to moderate or severer dementia, more information is needed regarding its sensitivity to different diagnostic areas.

Jacobs, Bernhard, Delgado, and Strain (1977) have proposed a quick mental status evaluation for use with medical patients. In this screen, the patient is asked questions regarding orientation to date and place (but not to person or time), questions requiring fundamental arithmetic operations, questions requiring immediate and delayed memory operations, and questions requiring the subject to supply synonyms and antonyms. There was no report of the test-retest reliability of this procedure; however, the interscorer reliability was reported to be 1.0 in an extremely limited sample of six subjects. Subjects who score less than 30 points should be suspected of organic impairment, and further evaluation is indicated.

ESSENTIALS OF THE EXTENDED MENTAL STATUS EXAMINATION

Remembering the variability of individuals can help keep the clinician from thinking that all clients with disorder X will exhibit symptoms Y and Z. Such a clinician not only misses the richness of clinical detail in each case, but also runs the risk of overlooking ancillary or seemingly unrelated symptoms and complaints.

To help the clinician organize his thoughts, observations, and procedures, the MSE can be conducted in a hierarchical fashion. For all of their diversity, modern theories of brain function share the notion of the brain as the locus of a system of interrelating cognitive processes that are organized in some form of a hierarchy. Starting at the simplest levels and working up through more complex levels can help streamline the procedure of assessment by ruling out certain areas for which their component skills have already been seen to be impaired. As an example, if the client is unable to add or subtract single digits in her head, the clinician does not need to assess the ability of the client to perform serial subtractions.

Level of Consciousness

The first area of brain function to be evaluated is the level of consciousness. If the client is able to appear for an outpatient appointment, a certain level of consciousness can be assumed. However, for the inpatient client, there is likely to be more variability in levels of consciousness. Although it is unlikely that psychologists who work in an outpatient clinic setting will see injured patients in the acute stages of their injury, this occurrence is much more likely for clinicians working in a hospital setting. Here, the attending physician may call for a consultation to help determine the level of cognitive functioning to obtain a baseline, to chart recovery, or to document level of functioning to aid in placement planning. Therefore, we start by discussing some of the methods for assessing lower levels of cognitive functioning and move upward in the hierarchy. There have been several systems for evaluating and reporting the level of consciousness. We review some of them subsequently.

Strub and Black (1993) suggest that the level of consciousness be classified according to a four-part Guttman-type scale. Patients are assigned to one or another of these categories by noting the patient's response to some form of stimulation. There is a wide range of possible stimulation techniques and a probably even wider range of patient responses. Therefore, it is important that the clinician document what form of stimulation was employed and what the response of the patient was. Relevant dimensions of patient response include eye openings and other eye movements, the presence of eye contact, the amount and quality of movement of any body parts, whether the patient engaged in speech and what the quality and content of that speech was, and a description of what the patient did following the assessment—whether he went back to sleep, asked for medication or food, and so forth.

In the first category, *Coma*, the client is not arousable. The client remains unconscious regardless of what the environmental stimulation may be. A client in this category will not respond to verbal stimulation or even to painful stimulation. An example of the clinician's documentation of such a case would be "Patient did not respond to my entering the room or calling out her name. No response to pinching the upper part of the shoulder. Patient appears to be in coma."

In the second category, *Semicoma* or *Stupor*, the patient is unconscious when the clinician enters the room and does not respond to verbal stimulation. The patient in this category will respond momentarily to persistent stimulation. Methods for eliciting a patient's response here can include shaking the patient's shoulder or pinching a fleshy part of the patient. An example of documentation would be "Patient responded to persistent shaking of his shoulder by mumbling and rolling over; did not regain consciousness."

In the third category, *Lethargy*, the patient will respond to stimulation, but only briefly before falling back to unconsciousness or sleep. An example of documentation would be "Patient responded to my calling out her name by briefly opening her eyes. She was able to answer one question before falling back to unconsciousness. Could be reawakened by calling her name again, but repeated the pattern of losing consciousness after a short period."

In the fourth category, *Alert*, the patient can respond to environmental stimulation. She is able to answer questions and to interact with others. For psychiatric patients, interaction with others will be moderated by level of motivation. Paranoid patients may have the capability to interact with others but may choose not to do so. The clinician's judgment is important in such cases.

There are multiple reasons why the patient may behave in a particular manner following stimulation by the clinician. For example, lethargy may be secondary to a recent dose of pain medication. The clinician should therefore note the time of day when assessment was conducted as well as the recent previous events. In inpatient settings, the nursing staff can be helpful in obtaining the relevant information.

The Glasgow Coma Scale

Another system of describing the level of consciousness is known as the Glasgow Coma Scale (Teasdale & Jennett, 1974), which we have already briefly discussed (see Table 1.5). The Glasgow Coma Scale was also developed as a Gutman-type scale. Patient responses are evaluated in three major areas, and the highest level of response for each area determines the Glasgow Coma score.

The first area of patient responses is that of motor responses. The highest level of response here is an ability to obey commands. The commands may vary along a continuum of difficulty and complexity, but should not be so simple as to be confused with a reflexive motor response. For example, when placing one's finger in the patient's hand, the patient may grasp the finger regardless of whether a verbal command to do so is given. Commands that are less likely to be confounded with reflexes include raising the arm, turning the head, or moving a major limb. Keeping in mind that such movements may also occur spontaneously, successfully completed commands should be repeated to assess the reliability of the results.

If the patient does not respond to verbal commands, one can apply a painful stimulus. One should be sensitive to whether any subsequent movement appears to be an attempt to move the limb from the painful stimulus or simply reflexive movement. The next lower level of motor response is the flexor response. In this response, the patient reacts to the clinician straightening her abducted limb by resuming abduction. The next lower level is extensor posturing, and the lowest level is no response.

Verbal responses constitute the second area of assessment in the Glasgow Coma Scale. At the top end of this scale the patient is able to state accurately his name, the place and why he is there, the city, year, month, date, and approximate time. Any inaccuracies in the patient's orientation should be noted.

The next lowest level of verbal responses is known as confused conversation. In this condition, the patient is able to respond verbally to questions and to keep her attention on the clinician, but the verbalizations of the patient indicate that she is confused about the situation or about the question of the examiner. For example, one of our head trauma patients was given the question, "What is your son's name?" to which he replied "1913." The patient was sitting up in bed, watching television, and appeared to be normal. Further questioning indicated that the patient thought that the soap opera on the television was some sort of game show for which he could not figure out the rules.

In the next lowest level of verbal responses, inappropriate speech, the client uses speech that is recognizable as words but that seems unrelated to environmental events. This speech appears to be random and is often loudly exclamatory or vulgar. In this level the patient is unable to conduct a conversation.

The next to lowest level of verbal response is that of incomprehensible speech. In this category, the patient will exhibit groaning or other sounds that do not have semantic referents. In the lowest level, there is no sound produced via the speech apparatus.

The third area of responses relates to eye opening. Spontaneous eye openings consistent with the patient's sleep/wake cycle is the highest level of response in this area. There are no assumptions made regarding the level of attention here or whether the patient is able to understand what is going on around her.

The next level of response in this category is eye opening in response to speech. Because of the difficulty in determining whether the patient is responding to a command to open the eyes or is merely responding to the verbal stimulation, the difference between the two is not scored here. The determination is made by whether or not the patient opens the eyes when speech, loud or otherwise, is produced by the clinician.

The next to last level is eye opening in response to pain. Here the painful stimulus is best applied at a site distant to the eye. Reflexive responses in the oscular muscles to the pain may otherwise obscure the nature of the response. The last level is, of course, no eye opening.

Rancho Los Amigos

Still another scale that has been used to describe levels of arousal is the Rancho Los Amigos Scale. Actually, the Rancho Los Amigos Scale attempts to describe levels of cognitive functioning. Rather than assessing the level of functioning separately in different areas as the Glasgow Coma Scale does, the Rancho Los Amigos Scale uses a unidimensional scale of generally increasing levels measured in different areas simultaneously. There are seven levels to this scale.

The first level is "No Response." Here the patient appears to be completely unresponsive to any stimulation. The second level is "Generalized Response." Here the patient may inconsistently react to stimuli. The reactions involve orientation responses and attempts to withdraw from a painful stimulus, but there is an absence of meaningful responses.

The third level is "Localized Response." Here the patient may react in a meaningful way to a stimulus, but the response is delayed and may be inconsistent. Simple commands may be followed, but, again, this occurs in an inconsistent manner. In the fourth level, "Confused-Agitated," the patient may exhibit a fairly high level of activity, but she does not appear to be able to process information meaningfully. Often, aggressive behavior is present. The patient does not discriminate between persons and objects. Verbalization occurs for the first time here, but it is incoherent or inappropriate. In this level, the patient is unable to care for herself, although motor activity such as rocking or pacing may be present.

The fifth level is "Confused, Inappropriate, Nonagitated." Here the patient is alert and can respond to simple commands consistently. However, she is unable to perform to complex commands. This patient is highly distractible and needs frequent redirection to remain on task. Memory is impaired, but the patient can usually recognize family members.

In the sixth level, "Confused-Appropriate," the patient demonstrates instrumental, means-ends behavior but requires external direction for successful completion of most complex tasks. He can follow simple commands. This patient is oriented to time and place. Memory is still somewhat impaired. He is able to perform most activities of daily life with minimal supervision.

The seventh level is "Automatic-Appropriate." Here the patient is able to perform most required activities but goes through the behaviors in a seemingly automatic fashion. This patient has superficial awareness of her condition and exhibits poor judgment. Some of these patients may be appropriate for vocational rehabilitation.

In the eighth and final level, "Purposeful and Appropriate," the patient is alert and oriented. He is able to learn new skills and is aware of his current condition. He is able to perform most activities independently.

From examining the preceding levels, it becomes clear that not all patients will fit neatly into one of the levels. Individuals may be in one level for a given area of functioning and in another level for a different area. However, as a gross indication of the level of functioning as well as of the extent to which independent functioning is possible, the Rancho Los Amigos Scale may be helpful.

ORIENTATION

Orientation is a term used to described the accuracy of a patient's perception and understanding of the events surrounding him. Orientation is not a unitary construct but is instead composed of different types. Commonly, these are referred to as orientation to person, place, date, and time. For most patients, these can be placed along a continuum of difficulty and seriousness with lack of orientation to person being the most serious and lack of orientation to time being the least serious. In most situations, orientation is assessed by simply asking the client her name, the place, the date, and the time. Orientation to the date can be further broken down into accuracy for year, season, month, day, and date. Despite its history as a usually informal assessment technique, there are a few standardized procedures available to assess orientation.

The Galveston Orientation and Amnesia Test (GOAT) was designed to evaluate orientation in head trauma patients and to chart changes as the recovery process progresssed (Levis, O'Donnell, & Grossman, 1979). The GOAT is very short and consists of only 10 basic questions that cover orientation to person, place, time, and date, as well as questions regarding memory for events directly preceding and following the injury. It is scored not only for whether the answers provided by the patient are correct but also for the degree of accuracy of the answer. For example, five error points are assigned if the subject is unable to recall what happened right before the injury occurred, and another five error points are assigned if the patient is unable to recall any events before the injury. The GOAT has been found to be related to Glasgow Coma Scale scores, to CT results, and to eventual recovery outcome of the patient. Normative data, based on a sample of 50 patients, is also available (Levin, O'Donnell, & Grossman, 1979).

Benton, Van Allen, and Fogel (1964) have standardized an instrument that can be used to assess temporal orientation in both inpatients and outpatients. In this evaluation, the patient is asked to state the current date, the day of the week, and the time of day. Scoring is performed by assigning each patient 100 points and subtracting points for each error made. One point is subtracted for day of the week for which patients are inaccurate (to a maximum of 3 points), 1 point is subtracted for each day of the month the patient is off (to a maximum of 15 points), and 5 points are subtracted for each month the patient is off (to a maximum of 30 points), with the exception that if the date is correct within 15 days, points are taken off for the date but not the month. For example, if the correct date is March 7 and the patient replies "February 27," points are subtracted for the incorrect date but not for the incorrect month. Ten points are subtracted for each year removed from the current year (to a maximum of 60 points), with the exception that if the patient response is within 15 days of the correct answer and the assessment occurs near the beginning or end of the year, no points are subtracted for the incorrect year. For example, if the date is January 12, 1988, and the subject replies "December 30, 1987," no points are subtracted for the year, although points are subtracted for the incorrect day. Finally, 1 point is subtracted for each $1/2$ hour for which the patient is incorrect (to a maximum of 5 points).

The differential weights assigned to types of errors indicate that this Test of Temporal Orientation is sensitive both to the presence of error as well as to the seriousness of the error. The performance of 110 medical inpatients without suspicion of organic mental impairment indicated that only 9 percent of the patients scored between 98 and 95 points, the remainder scoring higher. For the 60 cognitively impaired patients, 27% scored between 98 and 95 points, and 13% scored even lower. However, it must be pointed out that 458 of the cognitively impaired patients gave perfect scores on this assessment. Levin and Benton (1975) subsequently found that the Test of Temporal Orientation identified temporally disoriented patients about $1 1/3$ times as frequently as the standard neurological examination. Later Natelson, Haupt, Fleisher, and Gray (1979) reported that normal patients with lower amounts of education tended to make more errors than did normal patients with more education. In this sample, 5 percent of the normal medical patients achieved scores lower than 97. Unfortunately, the authors do not report the actual score distribution, so it is difficult to tell what the scores of those lower subjects were. However, it appears safe to say that scores lower than 95 should be an indication that a more thorough evaluation is in order. It is important to remember that because 45% of the impaired subjects in the original sample gave perfect scores, this screening test should not be used to rule out impairment but rather to indicate which patients are most appropriate for referral to a specialist. In general, significant disruption of orientation (i.e., year, month, and place) in the absence of a serious psychiatric disorder should be followed up with a more extensive MSE as eventual referral to a specialist.

ATTENTION

Once the level of consciousness has been assessed, the level of attention can be evaluated. Naturally, if the patient is unconscious, the assessment can terminate there. However, in the outpatient setting, attention is the first area likely to be assessed, especially if the patient is self-referred and the clinician is naive as to the condition of the patient. *Attention* is sometimes defined as the ability to attend to specific stimuli without distraction. The fact that the root (attend) is used in the definition speaks to the difficulty of defining such a term. Attending involves focusing one's perceptual mechanisms on a particular stimulus and actively processing the information. These are all private events. We can only assess attention by behavioral observation of the covert by-products of attention, by history, or by the use of procedures that require attention for their successful completion. An example of such procedures is the Digit Span portion of the WAIS-R. (Other examples will be given later in this section.)

Vigilance is another term that is often invoked in a discussion of attention. Vigilance is usually used to describe a sustained period of attention, such as attention for 30 seconds. Vigilance figures heavily in the experimental literature. There are many procedures for assessing vigilance in the laboratory. There are discrimination paradigms, reaction time paradigms, and others that are not easily duplicated in a clinical setting. However, there are several procedures that can be used to assess vigilance in the clinical setting.

One of these procedures is the "Random Letters Procedure." To use this procedure one must first have prepared a list of 75 letters in random order. One letter, say the letter *C*, should be repeated 10 times in the list. The clinician states the letters at the rate of three per 2 seconds and instructs the subject to tap a pencil each time she hears the letter *C*. Subjects with unimpaired vigilance should be able to make no more than one error in a 30-second period.

One method of assessing vigilance or sustained attention for shorter periods is to have the subject listen to a series of taps that the examiner makes under the table or that the examiner has prerecorded. It is important that the subject not receive extra cues from visual information. The series of taps should vary in length from 3 to 15. Have the subject count the taps and report the number. A normal subject should not have more than minimal trouble with this task.

Attention can be assessed throughout the MSE by observing the ability of the patient to follow the course of the examiner's verbalizations. For example, if the patient often has to request that the examiner repeat questions, it may be an indication that the patient is having difficulty maintaining sustained attention. If the patient replies to questions with inappropriate answers, the examiner should repeat the question to make sure that a receptive language impairment is not the responsible issue. For example, if in reply to the question, "How long have you lived at your current address?," the subject replies "297 Spruce Street," the examiner can repeat the question. If the subject now replies "About 2 years," the initial incorrect answer may reflect poor attention rather than a deficit in understanding verbal communication.

One aspect of attention relates to the ability of the subject to finish a mental operation that requires some thought. A procedure that can be used to assess this aspect is the use of serial subtractions. Tell the patient to start at 100 and subtract 7, then subtract 7 from that number, and so on. Serial subtractions is a complex activity that requires arithmetic ability and memory as well as mental control, so impaired performance may not be specifically related to impaired attention. However, if impairments in the other skill areas can be ruled out, impaired attention may be the cause of impaired performance. Assessing the qualitative components of performance can also help in interpreting results from this type of assessment. People with lower education levels may perform correctly but slowly. People with impaired arithmetic skills may perform at a reasonable rate, but their performance will be inaccurate. People with impaired attention will give a more variable performance. They will be slow and inaccurate. They may drift off, forgetting the task at hand. Or they may start the procedure, only to stop and ask the examiner what the question was.

Attention is also sometimes applied to the question of whether or not the subject is capable of attending to the entire perceptual field simultaneously. There are two general classes of disorders that impair this type of attention. The first, visual field cuts (sometimes called homonomous hemianopsia if the same side of the visual field is missing in each eye) are usually the result of a cerebral vascular accident. Unilateral neglect involves inattention to an entire side of one's perceptual field. These patients may read only the right side of a card with printed letters. In an extreme form of hemiinattention a patient familiar to us would dress only the right side of his body and would shave only the right side of his face. More often than not, a patient with this type of disorder will have a subtler presentation. Because of the strong contingencies usually present in the natural environment, people with this type of disorder will quickly develop compensating strategies such as alternate visual scanning procedures. Assessment of these suspected deficits can therefore be tested using double simultaneous stimulation.

In double simultaneous stimulation procedures, first unilateral sensory stimulation is confirmed. This is accomplished by presenting stimulation (e.g., visual, auditory, or tactile) to only one side of the body. After single sensory reception has been verified, both sides of the body are stimulated at the same time.

To test the visual fields, one stands about 3 feet in front of the patient and instructs the patient to fixate at the examiner's nose. The examiner then, spreading his arms and pointing his fingers inward, will wiggle one or the other, asking the subject which finger is being wiggled. The arms are moved in a general circle around the subject's face. If the subject is unable to state which finger is being wiggled correctly, the examiner moves the finger in, reducing the size of the visual field until the finger movement is recognized. The examiner should try to ascertain that the subject remains fixated on the examiner's nose during this procedure as lateral eye movements will invalidate the results. Finally, the examiner can alternate both fingers wiggling with only one finger moving to see if the subject can identify movement on both sides of the body at the same time. Failure on this task is referred to as *suppression* by the neuropsychologist and *extinction* by the neurologist. Suppressions can occur across different sensory modalities.

Auditory unilateral inattention is tested by standing behind the subject (out of the subject's line of sight), and lightly but audibly rubbing one's fingers close to the subject's ears. First one side is tested and then the other, and then both simultaneously. Again, the subject is asked to identify the correct side of the body being stimulated.

Tactile hemiinattention can be tested by lightly touching the cheek of a blindfolded subject with a cotton swab or the edge of a tissue, first one side and then the other, and, finally, both. Before using this procedure, it is important to first describe what will be done (i.e., "I am now going to touch you with the tip of a cotton swab"). This will help alleviate any anxiety caused by the blindfolding.

Deficits in unilateral attention are almost always the result of localized lesions in the cerebral cortex. Patients who demonstrate this type of deficit should be referred for a complete evaluation. Generalized inattention has a wider range of etiologies. Inattention may be caused by lesions in either the ascending or the descending reticular activation system. Alternatively, it may be the result of bilateral frontal lobe lesions. Either one of these will usually be accompanied by signs associated with the particular etiology, and diagnosis of one or the other should not be done on the basis simply of inattention. Inattention may also be the result of diffuse metabolic disorders. Uncontrolled diabetes, thyroid conditions, liver dysfunctions, and vascular disorders are only a few of the possible metabolic causes of inattention. Finally, disturbances in attention can also be the result of a psychiatric disorder such as depression or schizophrenia. The generalist clinician should not try to diagnose the problem, but should instead carefully document the observations made during the evaluation so as to be able to pass the information along to the specialist.

LANGUAGE

Language functions are required for the patient to understand and respond to questions by the examiner in all sections of the MSE. Therefore, the assessment of language functions is not confined to a separate section of the MSE, although there are particular procedures that can be used to assess language functions in this part of the evaluation. At a most general level, language functions can be dichotomized into receptive language function and expressive language functions. Receptive language skills include the ability to perceive and understand language whether it is communicated in an auditory/spoken modality or a written/visual modality. Expressive language skills also involve both auditory and written modalities. Further, both can be further be broken down into symbolic and sensory/motor aspects. In keeping with the proposed hierarchical structure of the MSE, the assessment of language functions starts at a simple level and progresses to a more complex level.

First, to assess comprehension, give the subject a series of simple commands progressing to more complex commands. This sequence may be useful.

1. Please close both of your eyes.
2. Now open both eyes.
3. Raise an arm.
4. Raise your left arm.

5. Put your right hand on your left knee.
6. If today is Tuesday, raise both of your arms; otherwise, raise only your right arm.

The earlier in this sequence that the subject fails, the more likely the need for a referral.

Assessing the level of expressive language functions includes testing the ability to name an object from a picture. It must be remembered that this sort of task (confrontation naming) is also affected by the general integrity of the visual system. Peripheral visual impairment as well as visual agnosia must be ruled out before an interpretation of expressive speech impairment is reached. The clinician can obtain pictures of everyday objects that can be readily recognized. Mount these singly on index cards. Present them one at a time to the patient and ask her to name the object pictured. Note whether the patient is able to state correctly the item or must instead describe its use. If the patient can name the object, note whether the pronunciation is correct. Keep in mind the regional differences in pronunciation that the patient might exhibit as a result of the location where the patient was raised. If the patient can neither name the object nor describe its use, she may have a visual agnosia, that is, an inability to recognize the meaning of visual information.

To assess the patient's basic levels of receptive and expressive language, one can start with a repetition task. Ask the patient to repeat what he hears. Give a list of words that progresses from short, simple words to more difficult words. For example, state, "Repeat after me— one, top, pipe, basket, cabinet, affection, stentorial, pleurisy, Methodist." Next, give the subject a card on which the same words have been printed and ask the subject to read them out loud. A differential between performance on the repetition task and the reading task can help determine the type of deficit involved. Any mispronunciations or stumbling should be noted.

If the patient is able to repeat and read simple words, move to phrases and finally sentences. The following phrases can be given orally first and then on a printed card.

1. In good time.
2. Follow the leader.
3. A ferocious lion.
4. Coming at an inconvenient time.
5. The boy kicked the ball.
6. The pitcher wound up and threw the ball.

7. If ever the sky should turn green, you should seek shelter.

Here the examiner should pay attention to elements of speech regulation as well as pronunciation. The ability to modulate speech tone may be impaired in some patients. These patients may demonstrate a monotone delivery, or, less commonly, may demonstrate abrupt and inappropriate changes in tone of voice.

To get an idea of the functional level of language skills, one can ask the patient to describe a picture that portrays more than one activity. Pictures of this sort can be found in popular news magazines and can be mounted on an index card. One can also ask the patient to describe his home (or job, hobby, or favorite television program). Here the clinician is attentive to multiple aspects of language production. If the patient has gotten this far in the evaluation of language, the more important aspects involve the ability to string together words in a manner that makes sense, appropriately matching the tone of voice to the content of the speech and speaking in a smooth manner. Additionally, the clinician should note the latency between giving the command and when the patient starts to reply as well as the relative richness or paucity of speech production. If there is low production, appropriate follow-up evaluation includes the use of the Controlled Oral Word Association Test or a vocabulary test.

The ability of the subject to write can also be assessed. Moving from simple words to simple phrases, the clinician can have the patient write from dictation and then copy from a printed card. The responses can be examined on the basis of spelling and legibility. Spelling errors should be evaluated in light of the patient's highest level of academic achievement. Legibility can be affected by motor problems that will be noticed in other parts of the MSE as well as here.

MEMORY

Memory impairment is a common complaint, both for patients with primarily psychological problems, such as depression and anxiety, and for patients with primarily neurological problems. Memory disruption is such a common complaint, it was at one time thought that all acquired brain impairment would include disturbances in memory. Many early screening tests for organic impairment were tests of memory. An example of this is the Wechsler Memory Scale (WMS). David Wechsler originally envisioned the WMS as a test for general organic impairment. Influenced by equipotentiality theory, he hypothesized that all head injuries would result in some memory impairment. There are other memory screening tests available, and those will be discussed in the section on screening instruments.

Memory is a multidimensional construct, and patients may be differentially impaired for different types of memory. Different researchers have proposed different subdivisions of memory. Among the most common are (1) verbal memory—memory for words, phrases, and short stories; (2) visual memory, memory for designs and colors; and (3) spatial memory—memory for the position of objects. Additionally, there may be memory for musical tones, tactile sensation, and proprioceptive information.

It is possible to obtain an informal assessment of memory within the confines of the MSE. Clinical evaluations of memory have tended to divide the assessment of memory into three categories: immediate memory, short-term memory, and long-term memory. These terms do not carry the same meanings in the clinical setting as they do in the laboratory investigations of memory and should not be confused with their laboratory and information processing meanings. In the clinical setting, *immediate memory* refers to events and occurrences in the MSE itself. *Short-term memory* refers to recent daily events. *Long-term memory* refers to remote events.

Short-term memory is usually assessed with a repetition task. In keeping with the preceding discussion regarding different types of memory, the clinician may want to assess the different types of memory separately. A prepared list of four unrelated words is useful in this evaluation. The examiner can give the list "violin, door, grape, pencil" and then ask the subject to repeat the list. This same list can be used to evaluate the effect of delay with distraction on memory. The clinician could then continue the evaluation. After 5 minutes have passed, the patient is again asked for the list of four words. Any four unrelated words can be used; however, it is a good idea to write down the list first to guard against the clinician forgetting the list or confusing it with a list used with another patient.

Some patients who are impaired for unrelated words may have normal memory when the verbal material is contained in a meaningful context, such as a short story. To assess this, the clinician can type a short story (similar to that used in the WMS) on an index card. Read the story to the patient and count the number of concepts in the story that the patient remembers. This assessment can again be conducted after 5 minutes to assess the effects of distraction and delay.

Still another type of memory involves the association of items. A card typed with a list of five related and unrelated pairs of words can be used in this evaluation. This procedure is similar to the Paired Associates section of the WMS and the Paired Words section of the Randt Memory Test. If the clinician is sure that neither of those two tests will be used in a later evaluation of the patient, those lists may be used here. However, it is more prudent to compose one's own unique list, so as not to bias and possibly invalidate later evaluations. A possible list is "opera–singer, railing–paper, dish–supper, cabinet–tiger, bell–ceiling." Both words are given at first, with pairs separated by a 1-second delay. Then only the first word is given, and the patient is asked to provide the second word. By repeating this procedure until the patient is able to state correctly each pair to a maximum of five trials, one can also assess the learning curve of the patient. Most normal subjects should be able to achieve a perfect score within three trials. The fact that some of the words are related and some are not will allow the clinician to assess informally differential memory for meaningful and nonmeaningful pairs. It should be remembered that this is an informal assessment without a normative base and no statements regarding a diagnosis of memory impairment without following the MSE with a standardized assessment.

Visual memory can be evaluated by showing the patient three pictures that can be clipped from a magazine and mounted on cardboard. The patient is then shown a series of six pictures, only three of which were included in the first series, and asked to identify which of the pictures he has seen before during the evaluation. Visual memory can also be assessed by showing the patient an abstract design such as in Figure 5-1. Allow the subject to view the design for 5 seconds. Then remove the design and ask the patient to draw the design. Impaired performance can be the result of problems in visual-motor coordination as well as in visual memory, so a report of the results should stick to a simple description of the behavioral task that the patient was unable to do.

Visual–spatial memory can also be assessed using a hidden objects procedure. In the presence of the subject, hide four objects. After a delay of 5 minutes, ask the patient to point out where the objects are hidden.

Recent memory is usually assessed by asking the patient about some events in his day, such as what he had for lunch, or what color the waiting room furniture was. The clinician should not ask questions for which she does not know the answer. Doing so would negate the purpose of the question. Long-term memory is usually assessed by asking the patient autobiographical questions, such as what was his childhood

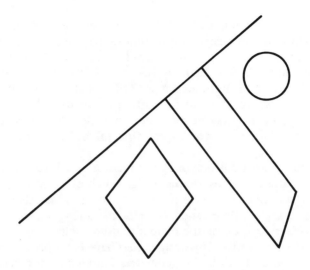

FIGURE 5.1 An example of a stimulus item that can be used for testing for visual memory.

home address, or what was the name of his fifth-grade teacher. Again, the clinician should know the correct answer for any questions asked. This can be accomplished by previously questioning a family member.

Impairment of immediate memory may be the result of lesions in the Sylvian fissure, or the result of a metabolic disorder, or the result of acute alcohol or drug intoxication. Disturbances of recent memory may be the result of subcortical lesions, especially lesions of the hippocampal region. Impairment of remote memory may be the result of frontal lesions or of diffuse cortical dysfunction. Transient global amnesia may result from TIAs and should be immediately followed up with a complete medical/neurological workup.

CONSTRUCTIONAL ABILITIES

The term *constructional abilities* refers to the ability to draw or build two- or three-dimensional objects. These require a complex combination of cortical-behavioral skills, and dysfunction in any one of the component skill areas can result in an impaired performance on a constructional task. Therefore, an impaired performance should be reported as such, and the generalist should resist the temptation to interpret the problem as a right-hemisphere lesion or a fine motor control dysfunction. Because of the complexity of skills required for successful performance, impairment of constructional abilities may be the early signs of a progressive disorder. Also chronic alcoholics and other substance abusers will sometimes show deficits in this area even when most other areas, particularly verbal skills, are intact. This occurs because in our culture verbal skills are the most highly practiced and overlearned. Although the general effect of substance abuse is not skill specific, decrements in performance will appear first in the least practiced skill areas.

Drawing to command is one method of assessing constructional abilities. Ask the patient to draw simple designs such as a circle, square, and triangle. If the patient is able to perform adequately, ask the patient to draw a more complex figure such as a clock showing a particular time. One traditional task is to ask the patient to draw a pipe.

Next ask the patient to copy designs that have been printed on index cards. These should include the geometric figures that the patient was earlier required to draw from command. The fact that a patient can draw from command, but cannot copy a design is important information in determining the type of deficit present.

In addition to drawing the three simple geometrical designs, the patient can be asked to copy a figure of a Greek cross, a horizontal diamond, a three-dimensional cube, or a three-dimensional pipe. The clinician should look for and report inaccuracies, distortions, and rotations of more than 45 degrees as these are all signs of organic impairment. Additionally, the patient may perseverate in drawing the design and draw more than one copy of the same stimulus, or he may fragment the design.

A method of assessing the spatial aspects of constructional deficits is to provide designs for the patient using pencils, tongue depressors, or blocks such as those used in the Koh's Block test or the Block Design subtest of the WAIS-R. When using the pencils or tongue depressors, first place one stick at a right angle to the edge of the table and ask the patient to replicate that design with a separate stick. Then place a stick parallel to the edge of the table with the same command. Next place two sticks at right angles to each other. Then place two sticks at a right angle to a third stick. Each time ask the patient to replicate the design. Here the clinician should pay attention to whether or not the patient is able to reproduce the angles. Not all normal patients will be able to reproduce the designs perfectly. However, deviations of more than 25 to 30 degrees should be noted and can be followed up by assessment with a short standardized instrument such as the Judgment of Line Orientation or the Visual Form Discrimination to determine the perceptual contributions.

As mentioned earlier, constructional dysfunctions can be the result of a multitude of organic etiologies. If the deficit is purely in spatial arrangement, it may the result of a right-hemisphere dysfunction. If the internal details of a reproduced design are disturbed, it may the result of a left-hemisphere dysfunction. Additionally, visual dysfunction may be the result of occipital dysfunction, deficits in visual integration may be the result of varietal dysfunction, and deficits in the direction of motor activity may be the result of frontal dysfunction. The general clinician should not try to diagnose these problems but should refer the patient to a specialist.

HIGHER COGNITIVE FUNCTIONS

Higher cognitive functions are those activities that require integration among different skill areas, the symbolic manipulation of information, abstract problem solving, planning, and judgment. There are many different cortical-behavioral skill areas that are involved in the successful completion of these tasks. As a result, if a patient shows impairment in the previously assessed skill areas, she is likely to demonstrate impaired performance in higher cognitive functions as well. It is also possible that patients who perform adequately in the earlier cortical-behavioral skill areas may not perform adequately in these skill areas. Especially in the early stages of a progressive dementia, the basic cognitive functions may maintain their integrity while the higher order cognitive functions may begin to break down.

It is also because of the complexity of these higher order functions that impaired performance may be exhibited by individuals with metabolic disorders, viral infections, or psychiatric disorders, especially thought disorders. So far we have strongly emphasized that the generalist clinician should not perform diagnosis using these procedures. This is of paramount importance in the case of the individual who exhibits deficits only in higher order cognitive functions. Even for the specialist, diagnosis of the individual who exhibits deficits solely in higher order functions is problematic. Cut-off scores are not always a useful index in these situations, and the interpretation of results relies on the consideration of qualitative aspects of the individual's performance.

For example, performance on higher order tasks is related to a large extent on the education and experience of the individual. This is true to a certain extent for most neuropsychological functions. However, it is less true for simple sensory functions than it is for abstraction tasks. Although it may not represent a serious problem if an individual with a history of an eighth-grade education is unable to state how a fox and a dog are alike, if a college-educated individual cannot perform the same task, it does represent a serious problem and a probable decline in abstraction skills.

The informal assessment of higher cognitive functions includes sampling the patient's fund of knowledge, the ability of the individual to manipulate old knowledge, the level of the individual's social awareness and judgment, and abstract thinking. The informal assessment will include procedures similar to procedures used in the Information, Similarities, and Arithmetic section of the WAIS-R. Because the patient is likely to receive the WAIS-R eventually, it is not a good idea to take procedures and questions directly from the WAIS-R or from other standardized assessment instruments. The clinician should instead formulate her own set of similar items with different content. Examples of such similar items include the following:

Similiarities
How are a bucket and a coffee mug alike? (A good response is, "They both can hold liquid"; a borderline response is. "They're both round.")
How are a bed and a couch alike? (A good response is, "They're both furniture"; a borderline response is, "They both have four legs," or "You can sleep on both of them.")

General Information
Why should people make out a will? (To avoid tax problems for beneficiaries and to make sure that your estate goes to the people you prefer.)

Why are blood tests required before marriage? (To screen for disease and check for possible Rh factor incompatibilities.)

Abstract Reasoning and Interpretation of Proverbs
What does this saying mean: Don't count your chickens before they are hatched? (One should not count on something before it happens.)

What does this saying mean: You have to sleep in the bed you made? (People have to face the consequences of their behavior.)

Another good way to test higher order cognitive functioning is to evaluate the ability of the person to finish a conceptual series. This task will help the clinician to obtain an informal assessment of the abstract reasoning ability of the patient. For this procedure, the clinician should prepare index cards with one series of symbols on each card. Show the series to the patient and ask what comes next.

What comes next in this series?
BDFHJ_____ (L)
11, 8, 5, _____ (3)
fire, 4, strut, 5, ox, 2, real, _____ (4)

COMPLEX FUNCTIONS

There are other complex functions that do not fit a well into our schema of cognitive skill areas. These functions can be readily assessed in the MSE. One of these miscellaneous areas involves what is called left-right confusion. In this condition the patient is unable to distinguish left from right reliably. Assessing this corticobehavioral skill is simply a matter of giving the patient verbal commands which require a knowledge of left and right for their successful completion. Start with easy commands, and if the patient is able to respond correctly, move on to more complex commands. For example, start by asking the patient to point to her right eye. Then ask the patient to touch his left shoulder with his left hand. Then ask the patient to point to your left hand. Finally, ask the patient to point to your right ear with her left hand.

A rare condition associated with lesions in the left parietal lobe is known as *finger agnosia*. In this condition the patient is unable to name the fingers of his hand. This can be assessed by asking the patient to point to your left middle finger. Show the patient one of your fingers and ask the name. Finally, blindfold the patient and lightly touch one of her fingers, asking the name of the finger.

CONCLUSIONS

As discussed earlier, the MSE is best conducted in a hierarchical fashion. Mental operations are complex combinations of component skills. When this fact is kept in mind, the assessment of mental operations can be conducted more efficiently. The organization of this chapter reflects current conceptions of the hierarchical organization. It is best to start by assessing the basic levels of arousal and orientation, moving through the assessment of attention, language, memory, constructional abilities, higher order cognitive functions, and, finally, the complex functions.

At each stage, failure of the patient to perform adequately has implications for the assessment of the following areas. Extremely poor performance in an early part of the MSE may indicate that the evaluation can be safely terminated. Naturally, if a patient is unconscious, the evaluation will be short. However, there are other points at which continuing the evaluation may be unnecessary. For example, if a patient demonstrates severe deficits in receptive language skills, poor performance on later sections of the MSE may not contribute further information. This is because the poor performance is likely to be due to an inability of the subject to understand what is required of him rather than an impairment in the specific skill area.

Conversely, if impairment in an early part of the MSE is only moderate, continuing the evaluation may add useful information. For example, if a patient demonstrates mild deficits in receptive language, the evaluation of constructional abilities may be conducted through the use of pantomime and example.

The flexibility of the MSE increases its efficiency in uncovering information. Because the clinician can also further assess skill areas for which the patient demonstrated problematic performance, the flexibility also increases the power of the MSE. Continued experience with the use of the MSE coupled with more extensive readings can help improve the ability of the clinician to use the MSE. This chapter should be viewed as only the beginning in learning to use the MSE to assess the possibility of organic impairment.

6

Screening Tests of Perceptual and Motor Functions

Until recently, most research conducted in neuropsychology has been directed toward the differentiation of the brain-damaged patient from all other patients. This research has focused on developing either a single test or a battery of tests that have the ability to make this discrimination. In a number of settings, the need exists for comprehensive neuropsychological evaluations to determine whether cortical dysfunction exists, as well as the extent and nature of the dysfunction; in using the results of the evaluation, there is a need for prediction of the best plan of rehabilitation.

In some situations, however, the clinician has the responsibility of assessing unselected cases to identify areas where additional evaluation is necessary. This generally occurs in psychiatric hospitals, rehabilitation facilities, mental health clinics, or private practice situations where psychological screening is routine with each patient. In these settings, examiners and clinicians usually do not choose to use a lengthy test battery because of the time and expense involved. A complete neuropsychological evaluation can routinely take 6 or more hours, and the initial materials can cost as much as $2400. Many psychiatric hospitals and mental health clinics have neither the personnel nor the space to devote to such lengthy examination procedures. This is particularly true in instances in which the base rate of neurological dysfunction is low in the population being screened. In these settings, a neuropsychological screening can be used effectively and efficiently to identify those individuals whose cases would be clarified through the use of more comprehensive examinations.

The screening examination is not an end in itself, because the conclusions obtained are quite limited. Rather, the clinician can determine whether the possibility of neuropsychological dysfunction exists. The screening tests and batteries that will be discussed in this section will not be able to identify the nature of a given disorder or the primary deficits in the patient's functioning. Nor can such an examination provide a reliable aid for treatment and rehabilitation.

The clinician who uses screening devices can use one of two approaches. First, he may employ a variety of tests that are highly sensitive to brain damage in general. Second, he can use a small battery of tests that can be analyzed in much the same fashion as a larger, more comprehensive test battery. The tests in such a battery need to be selected so that each is sensitive to a different type of dysfunction rather than the more global tests most appropriate for the first technique. All of the procedures that will be mentioned here are more sensitive to one kind of brain damage than to another. Thus the tests selected for a screening must complement each other, with as little redundancy as possible.

The remainder of this book, therefore, will concentrate on two basic types of instruments. The remainder of this chapter, as well as Chapters 8 and 9, deal with individual tests that have been shown to be sensitive to cognitive dysfunction; chapter 10 discusses some experimental batteries that have been used with success to identify the presence of brain damage. Finally, this chapter discusses recently introduced devices, both experimental and commercially available, designed to screen individuals for brain dysfunction.

VISUAL FUNCTIONS

There are a variety of aspects of visual functioning that can be impaired by brain dysfunction. As a general rule, brain damage that leads to the disruption of one visual function will affect a cluster of related visual functions as well. A major division in visual functions occurs between those involving verbal-symbolic material and those dealing with nonsymbolic stimuli. Other stimulus dimensions that may highlight different aspects of visual perception are the degree to which the stimulus is structured, the amount of remote and new memory involved in the task, spatial relationships, and the presence of interfering information. We will start with tests for the more basic functions, such as simple perception and recognition, and progress to higher-order tasks, such as visual-spatial relationships.

Color Perception

A screening test of color perception can serve a dual purpose in the assessment of patients in whom brain dysfunction is suspected. It can identify individuals with congenitally defective color vision (color blindness) whose performance on tasks requiring accurate color recognition might otherwise be misinterpreted. Such knowledge will have a significant impact on the clinician's overall interpretation of patient responses to such colored material as that in the Color Sorting Test and the Rorschach. Tests of color perception can also be used to determine the potential presence of color agnosia.

Two of the most widely used tests of color perception in a standard neuropsychological assessment are the Ishihara (1964) and the Dvorine (1953) Screening Tests. Each test requires that the patient view a card printed with different colored dots that form recognizable figures against a background of contrasting colored dots. All of the dots are matched for color saturation so that patient responses are not influenced by the "brightness" of a particular color. Those individuals who truly have defective color perception, and not a problem with color agnosia (the inability to identify colors despite intact color discrimination vision), will be unable to see the stimulus figure against the background. In contrast, those patients with intact color vision and a color agnosia will be able to make the discriminations necessary but may not be able to differentiate between a red ball and a blue ball.

The Color Perception Battery (De Renzi & Spinnler, 1967) is also a useful device. The test includes the Ishihara plates as well as tests of color matching, pointing to color, color drawing, color naming, and memory for colors. The purpose of this instrument is the discrimination of those individuals whose difficulty arises from purely perceptual deficits from those with a language component (aphasia) from those patients with other forms of the loss of knowledge about object colors.

VISUAL RECOGNITION

Interest in visual recognition has grown with the rapid expansion of knowledge of the different roles played by the hemispheres and with more precise understanding of the different functional systems within the brain. When brain damage is present or suspected, examining different aspects of visual recognition on a gross level can lead to a clearer idea of the patient's status. Assessment of visual processing is probably the most technically difficult of all areas of assessment (Beaumont & Davidoff, 1992). Visual processing deficits can cover numerous dimensions including location, size, brightness, contrast, movement, color, complexity, and sequence. In most instances, the general clinician will have neither the specialized training nor the equipment required to perform this type of assessment. However inadequate it may be methodologically, the clinician will typically be limited to a simple confrontational assessment of the visual fields, leaving detailed examinations to others—specially trained neuropsychologists (not all neuropsychologists have been adequately trained for this) and others who can perform psychophysical assessments.

Word Recognition

The typical comprehensive neuropsychological test battery or screening battery will generally include an assessment of word recognition, because defective word recognition is considered to be a predominant symptom in aphasia. However, there are two tests that can be useful when evaluating a nonaphasic patient for the presence of brain damage. *Patients with visual field defects, whether or not aphasia is present, tend to ignore the part of a printed line or long printed word that falls outside the range of their intact visual fields when the eyes are fixated for reading.* This can occur despite of the senselessness of what is read by the patient. Left hemisphere injury can cause the individual to ignore the right side of the printed material. This condition shows up readily on tasks of oral reading in which sentences are several inches long. Because the length and size of the stimulus material are important features, a newspaper article will not work because the size of the print and the width of the columns are too small. One method to test effectively for this phenomenon has been developed by Battersby and his associates. A set of ten cards was developed on which were printed 10 familiar four-word phrases in large letters (1 "high and 1/16" in line thickness). Omissions and distortions of the words is considered evidence of a visual field defect (Battersby, Bender, Pollack, & Kahn, 1956).

Picture Recognition

Meaningful Pictures (Battersby et al., 1956) was developed to bring out asymmetrical perceptual defects. The test requires a number of colored magazine illustrations or photographs that are essentially symmetrical on either side of the median plane. Each picture is presented first as a verbal recall task in which, after a 10-second exposure, the patient is asked to name and indicate the relative position of the details of the picture seen. When the recall section of the test is completed, the patient is again shown the illustration and asked to describe all its details while actually looking at it. Card sides can then be compared for the number of responses elicited from the patient. A preponderance of responses that describe one side of the picture or the other suggests the presence of lateralized visual inattention (or a lesion in the brain) on the opposite side.

Another commonly used test that can be used to assess visual recognition is the revised version of the Peabody Picture Vocabulary Test (PPVT) (Dunn & Dunn, 1981). The PPVT was designed primarily to assess an individual's receptive vocabulary. As such it is an effective tool for assessing aspects of both aphasia and perceptual functions. In the standard administration of the test, the patient is shown a series of pages, each of which has four pictures on it. The patient is required to indicate which of the four pictures on a given page best shows a word spoken by the examiner. The patient's response can be either verbal or gestural. A raw score is then calculated in terms of the total number of correct responses, which can then be converted into a number of standard or derived scores based on a large normative data base. A nonstandard administration used by some clinicians involves having the patient name a number of pictures on various pages. Although no normative or research data exist for this nonstandard administration, the patient's performance can give the clinician a fairly good idea as to whether a picture recognition deficit exists, from which the presence of possible brain dysfunction can be inferred.

Face Recognition

Barrington and James (1967) demonstrated that *there is no regular relationship between the inability to recognize familiar faces (prosopagnosia) and impaired recognition of unfamiliar faces.* This led to a separation of facial recognition tests into those that involve a memory component and those that do not. Tests of familiar facial recognition require a memory component and generally use the faces of popular figures and well-known historical figures; the memory element is one of the difficulties with this form of test. If a patient performs poorly on such a test, it is quite difficult to determine if the primary problem involves perceptual recognition or visual memory.

To avoid this difficulty and examine the ability to recognize faces without involving memory, Benton and Van Allen (1968) developed the Test of Facial Recognition. In this test, the patient is asked to match identical front-view photographs of an unknown person, front with side views, and front views taken under different lighting conditions. The test calls for 54 separate matches. The creators of the test have defined scores of 35 and 36 (correct) as "raising the question of possible cognitive dysfunction and scores below 33 . . . as indicating severe impairment" (Benton & Van Allen, 1972, p. 11).

A patient with problems in facial recognition usually will have right hemisphere dysfunction. Neither visual field defects nor the presence of aphasia will affect visual recognition scores (Lezak, 1983); however, facial recognition deficits do tend to occur with spatial agnosia and dyslexia, as well as with dysgraphias (problems with writing) that involve spatial disturbance (Tzavaras, Hecacn, & Le Bras, 1970).

Figure and Design Recognition

Simple Recognition

Perceptual recognition of meaningless designs is generally tested by having the subject draw a variety of designs from memory or from model figures. When a patient's design reproductions contain the essential elements of the original from which they were copied and preserve the proper interrelationships with general accuracy, the patient's perception has been adequately demonstrated (Lezak, 1983). The capacity to recognize meaningful information can be rapidly assessed using the first few pictures of the WAIS Picture Recognition suggest.

There are a number of other techniques to assess simple perceptual recognition. A very low level test of visual recognition can be found in the Discrimination of Forms subtlest of the Stanford-Binet (age level IV). The patient is shown 10 line drawings of common geometric figures (such as a square, circle, etc.), one at a time, and asked to point out the matching figure on a card on which all 10 figures are displayed. The first 12 items of the Raven's Progressive Matrices (Raven, 1960) can also be used as a test of simple recognition ability (Knehr, 1965).

There are also several devices that have been developed to ascertain intact perceptual closure including the Street Completion Test (Street, 1931), the Mooney Closure Test (Mooney & Ferguson, 1951), and the

Gestalt Completion Test (Ekstrom, French, Harman, & Dermen, 1976). The research conducted to date with these tests indicates that while they do effectively discriminate patients from controls, there are poor intercorrelations among these tests for non–brain-injured individuals (Wasserstein, 1980). Beaumont and Davidoff (1992) report that the Gollin Incomplete Figures (Gollin, 1960) is a useful instrument to assess recognition. The test comprises 20 sets of stimuli, each set of which is a progressively more complete representation of the object ranging from minimally to maximally recognizable. The test appears to assess the ability to extract perceptual features and is not especially sensitive to right posterior varietal lesions (Warrington & Rabin, 1970).

COMPLEX VISUAL FUNCTIONS—TESTS OF SPATIAL ABILITIES

Tests of complex visual abilities have long been popular as single tests of brain injury. This popularity appears to be based on the known representation of complex spatial functions in both cerebral hemispheres (Golden, 1981).

Bender Visual-Motor Gestalt

The Bender Visual-Motor Gestalt Test is probably the oldest test of complex visual processing. It is also arguably the most widely used single test of visual functioning. *The Bender-Gestalt is also the most widely misused test for determining the presence or absence of brain damage.* Several clinicians have a tendency to use the Bender, and only the Bender, to identify possible cortical dysfunction. This approach should be avoided, because the Bender Visual-Motor Gestalt has *not* been shown effectively to perform this exclusive function. The danger of this use lies in the Bender's high rate of false negative findings in uncovering general cortical dysfunction.

In using the Bender, the clinician asks the patient to copy nine geometric figures and patterns on a blank sheet of paper (see Figure 6.1). The drawings are then evaluated by one of several scoring systems that have been developed over the years. Each of these scoring systems has attempted to identify qualitative signs indicating brain damage. In some cases, variations of these scoring approaches also attempt to identify emotional disorders. The most popular of these scoring systems include

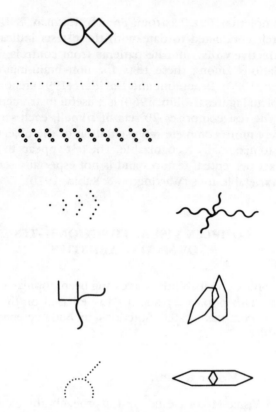

FIGURE 6.1   The Hutt adaptation of the Bender-Gestalt figures.
From Hutt, M. (1977). *The Hutt adaptation of the Bender-Gestalt Test.* New York: Grune
& Stratton. Reprinted by permission.

those presented by Bender (1938), Hain (1964), Hutt, (1969), and Pascal
and Suttell (1951).

Investigators who have used these scoring systems have reported up
to 70% accuracy in identifying brain-injured individuals and a hit rate of
90% in identifying normal subjects (e.g., Brilliant & Gynther, 1963;
Levine & Feirstein, 1972; Tymchuk, 1974). However, *there have been a
number of other studies using the Bender that have reported essentially negative results, particularly in those situations where the differentiation between brain-damaged and psychiatric patients was required* (Johnson, Hellkamp, & Lottman, 1971; Mosher & Smith, 1965;
Watson, 1968). Several major review articles have criticized the Bender

Visual-Motor Gestalt Test for its unreliability and inability to discriminate in psychiatric populations. Studies using the Bender have also received a good deal of criticism for not using control subjects (Billingslea, 1963; Canter, 1976; Tolor & Schulberg, 1963).

The results of this research indicate that the use of the Bender by itself allows far too wide a margin for error in clinical work. A poor score on the Bender may indeed indicate problems for a client; however, it does not specify the nature of the patient's problems. Similarly, and perhaps more importantly, a good score on the Bender does not rule out the possibility of the presence of brain damage. The Bender does its job well as a visual-perceptual screening device when it is used in conjunction with other tests. It should never be used as the sole index of brain damage when screening a patient for the presence of cortical dysfunction.

Difficulties on the Bender are more likely to appear with varietal lobe deficits (Garron & Cheifetz, 1965); of these, lesions in the right parietal region have been associated with the poorest performances (Biller, Ben-Yishay, Gerstman, Goodkin, Gordon, & Weinberg, 1974). *Distortions are the errors most likely to be associated with organicity. Rotation occurs with both right and left hemisphere lesions, but about twice as often in the presence of right-sided damage.*

The clinician is cautioned that these results pertain largely to adults. We mention this because the Bender is also very widely used in the assessment of children. Poor performance of a child on the Bender Visual-Motor Gestalt Test is interpreted differently from that of an adult, and a different scoring approach is used.

Background Interference Procedure for the Bender Visual-Motor Gestalt

This procedure developed from Arthur Canter's observation that distraction on the Bender-Gestalt response sheet (a coffee stain) impaired the performance of brain-injured patients more than other patients (Golden, 1981). The test requires that the patient draw the nine Bender figures on a blank sheet of paper and then draw them a second time on a sheet of paper printed over with a series of irregular wavy lines. The procedure assumes that the interference caused by the wavy lines will be most disruptive for individuals with brain damage. The scoring system employs a modification of Pascal and Suttell's (1951) Bender scoring system (Canter, 1976). The score on the standard administration of the Bender is subtracted from the score obtained on the interference administration to yield a measure of the effect of the interference.

Research indicates a hit rate of approximately 88% (Canter, 1976; Golden, 1981). Using an older scoring system for the test, Canter (1966) reported a 73% success rate in differentiating brain-damaged from psychotic patients. Subsequent replications, using the interference procedure, have reported higher hit rates (Canter, 1971, 1976). The procedure appears to have a reasonably high reliability, up to 0.9 in some cases (Adams, 1966; Canter, 1976; Song & Song, 1969).

Memory for Designs

This test is similar to other drawing tests, except that the designs must be drawn from memory (Graham & Kendall, 1960). While the memory aspect introduces another component to the testing situation, the test is quite effective, as will be seen, and therefore should be considered when deciding on specific tests to use during a screening examination for brain damage. The scoring system for the test penalizes rotations and other errors common to the Bender-Gestalt scoring systems more than it does losses in memory. Consequently, the test yields a score that can be considered comparable to those obtained on the Bender Visual-Motor Gestalt (Quattlebaum, 1968).

Correct classification rates of 63% for brain-damaged individuals and 88 % for psychiatric controls have been reported in one study (Brilliant & Gunther, 1963). A number of other studies have also reported positive results in the same range of effectiveness as for the Bender (e.g., McManis, 1974; Shearn, Berry, & Fitzgibbons, 1974). It should be noted, however, that Black (1974) reported that the Memory for Designs Test was not at all effective in discriminating patients with mild frontal lobe injuries. Also, Watson (1968) reported that the test was unable to differentiate between chronic schizophrenics and brain-injured individuals.

Benton Visual Retention Test

The Benton Visual Retention Test (BVRT) consists of three alternate but equivalent versions that may be administered under differing conditions (Benton, 1973; Sivan, 1991). The conditions include simple copying and copying from memory after various delays (no delay and 15-second delay). Each version of the test consists of 10 cards with more than one figure in the horizontal plane; most have three figures, two large and one small, with the small figure always at one side or the other. In addition to visual memory, the test is sensitive to disruptions in visual-spatial processing.

Each version of the test is scored for both the number of correct designs and the number of errors. Six types of errors are possible: omissions, distortions, perseverations, rotations, misplacements (in the relative positioning of one figure to the others), and errors in size. Therefore, it is common to have more than one error per card. Both the number correct and the error score norms for Administration A (the most frequently used administration consisting of a 10-second exposure and then immediate copying from memory) take into account intelligence level and age as shown in Table 6.1.

Interpretation of the test results is relatively straightforward. Taking the age and level of intellectual functioning of the patient into account, the clinician uses the normative tables for Administration A and determines whether either score (number correct or number of errors) falls into the impaired range. Benton (1974) considers a score of 2 points below the number of expected correct responses to "raise the question of impairment," whereas 4 or more points below the expected score is viewed as a "strong indication" of impairment. Error scores are dealt

TABLE 6.1 BVRT Norms for Administration A: Adults Expected Number of Correct Scores and Error Scores by Estimated Premorbid IQ and Age

Estimated premorbid IQ	Expected no. correct by age		
	15–44	45–54	55–64
110 and up (superior)	9	8	7
95–109 (average)	8	7	6
80–94 (low avg.)	7	6	5
70–79 (borderline)	6	5	4
60–69 (mild MR)	5	4	3
59 and lower (MR)	4	3	2

	Expected no. errors by age			
	15–39	40–54	55–59	60–64
110 and up (superior)	1	2	3	4
105–109 (high avg.)	2	3	4	5
95–104 (average)	3	4	5	6
90–94 (low avg.)	4	5	6	7
80–89 (dull avg.)	5	6	7	8
70–79 (borderline)	6	7	8	9
60–69 (mild MR)	7	8	9	10
59 and below (MR)	8	9	10	11

Source: Lezak, M.D. (1976). *Neuropsychological assessment.* Nenv York: Oxford University Press. Copyright © 1976, Oxford University Press. Adapted by permission.

with in a similar fashion. A patient whose error score exceeds the expected score, based on age and intelligence, by 3 or more points can be suspected of being impaired, and an error score exceeding the expected level by 5 or more points is considered a "strong indication" of brain dysfunction. Similar scoring criteria and methods are used for the other versions of the BVRT.

Errors on the BVRT can also be tabulated by type, enabling the clinician to determine the nature of the patient's problem. Lezak (1983) notes that impaired immediate memory or an attention disorder appear mostly as a simplification, simple substitution, or omission of the designs. Unilateral spatial neglect tends to appear as a consistent omission of the figure on the same side of the design. Practice deficits most often manifest as defects in the execution or organization of the drawings. Rotations and consistent design distortions generally indicate a more basic perceptual problem. Perseverations should alert the clinician to look elsewhere in the patient's testing protocol for other perseverations on different tasks. Widespread perseveration may suggest a monitoring or activity control problem, whereas perseveration limited to performance on the BVRT is usually indicative of a specific visual or immediate memory impairment in a patient who is trying hard to compensate for, or cover up, brain dysfunction. Simplification of designs, including a disregard of size and figure placement, has been associated with a generalized behavioral regression (Lezak, 1983).

There is a good deal of evidence to suggest that the BVRT, when compared with other single tests, is rather effective in discriminating groups of patients with brain damage from groups with psychiatric disorders (Fenton, 1974; Brilliant & Gynther, 1963). It is not accurate enough, however, to be used singly for individual diagnostic decisions (Watson, 1968). As with other tests of visual functioning, patients with right hemisphere lesions tend to perform more poorly than do patients with left-sided brain damage. In addition, *patients with more posterior damage (in the parietal-occipital region) do Snore poorly than do those with more anterior dysfunction*. The clinician must remain cognizant of the fact that the above statements reflect only statistical associations and are not hard-and-fast rules for diagnosis from BVRT results. The BVRT-R (Sivan, 1991) features updated and expanded normative data, as well as a reasonably detailed review of research conducted with the test. Of note is the vastly improved format of the response record, which make recording and scoring of the test a good deal easier than was the case previously. Also, the test publisher has included a scoring template that assists in the scoring of the more detailed aspects of the individual reproductions.

Rey-Osterrieth Complex Figure Test

A "complex figure" was devised by Rey (1941) to investigate both perceptual organization and visual memory in brain-damaged individuals. Osterrieth (1944) standardized Rey's procedure and obtained normative data from the performance of 230 normal children, with ages ranging from 4 to 15, and 60 adults in the 16-to-60 age range. He also gathered data from a small group of adults (43) who had sustained traumatic brain damage, as well as from a few patients with endogenous brain disease.

The test consists of Rey's figure (see Figure 6.2), two blank sheets of paper, and five or six colored pencils. The patient is first asked to copy the figure, which has been placed so that its length runs along the pa-

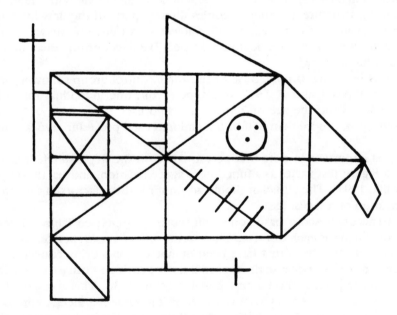

FIGURE 6.2 Rey-Osterrieth Complex Figure Test.
From Osterrieth, P.A. (1944). Le test de copie d'une figure complex. *Archives de Psychologie, 30,* 224. Reprinted by permission.

tient's horizontal plane. The examiner watches the performance closely. Each time a section of the figure is completed, a different-colored pencil is handed to the patient, and the order of colors is recorded. Time needed to complete the figure is noted, and both the figure and drawing are removed from the patient's field of vision. After 3 minutes, the subject is given a second sheet of paper and is asked to draw the design from memory. The time to complete the drawing is recorded, as is whether the patient follows the same procedural approach on the second drawing as on the first.

Osterrieth analyzed the drawings in terms of the patient's method of procedure as well as specific copying errors. Seven procedural types were identified. (1) Subject begins by drawing the large central rectangle and details are added in relation to it. (2) Subject begins with a detail attached to the central rectangle, or with a subsection of the rectangle, completes the rectangle, and adds remaining details in relation to the rectangle. (3) Subject begins by drawing the overall contour of the figure without explicit differentiation of the central rectangle and then adds internal details. (4) Subject juxtaposes details one by one without an organizing structure. (5) Subject copies discrete parts of the drawing with no semblance of organization. (6) Subject substitutes the drawing of a similar object, such as a boat or a house. (7) Subject produces an unrecognizable drawing.

In Osterrieth's sample, 83% of the adult control group followed procedure types 1 and 2, 15% used type 4, and one individual followed type 3. Beyond the age of 7 years, no child used types 5, 6, or 7, and from age 13, more than half of the children used procedure types 1 and 2.

It is important to note that performance on the Rey-Osterrieth Complex Figure Test varies as a function of age, education, and sex (Roselli & Ardila, 1991). The clinician should account for these factors in the interpretation of test results.

An accuracy score, based on a unit scoring system (see Table 6.2), can be obtained for each test trial. The scoring units refer to specific areas or details of the figures that have been numbered for scoring convenience (see Figure 6.3). Because the reproduction of each unit can earn as many as 2 score points, the highest possible score is 36. The average adult scores 32. The memory trial is scored in the same manner. A comparison of the scores for each trial will aid the clinician in determining the presence of visuographic or visual-memory defects, as well as their relative severity (Table 6.3). As such, the use of this test can supplant using the Bender and BVRT because comparable information is obtained.

TABLE 6.2   Scoring System for the Rey-Osterrieth Complex Figure Test

Units

1.   Cross upper left corner, outside of rectangle
2.   Large rectangle
3.   Diagonal cross
4.   Horizontal midline of 2
5.   Vertical midline
6.   Small rectangle, with 2 to the left
7.   Small segment above 6
8.   Four parallel lines within 2, upper left
9.   Triangle above 2, upper right
10.   Small vertical line within 2, below 9
11.   Circle with 3 dots within 2
12.   Five parallel line with 2 crossing 3, lower right
13.   Sides of triangle attached to 2 on right
14.   Diamond attached to 13
15.   Vertical line within triangle 13 parallel to right vertical of *a*
16.   Horizontal line within 13, continuing 4 to right
17.   Cross attached to lower center
18.   Square attached to 2, lower left

Scoring

Each of the eighteen units above is considered separately. Each unit is scored
for accuracy and relative position within the whole of the design.
For each unit, count as follows:

Correct _____	Placed properly _____	2 points
_____	Placed poorly _____	1 point
Distorted or incomplete _____	Placed properly _____	1 point
but recognizable _____	Placed poorly _____	½ point
Absent or not recognizable _____		0 points
Maximum possible score _____		36 points

Source: Lezak, M.D. (1976). *Neuropsychological assessment.* New York: Oxford University
Press. Copyright © 1976, Oxford University Press. Adapted by permission.

Perceptual Maze Test

The Perceptual Maze Test, developed by Elithorn (1955), is based on his
view that "perceptual skills are phylogenetically fundamental components of intelligent behavior." In this test, the patient must find a path-
way through a series of dots distributed on a triangular grid. The number of correct routes possible is limited because the route selected must
pass through a specific number of dots and progress steadily toward the
top of the grid along fixed diagonals. The test is scored on the basis of a
1-minute time limit, of which the patient is not to be informed. Each

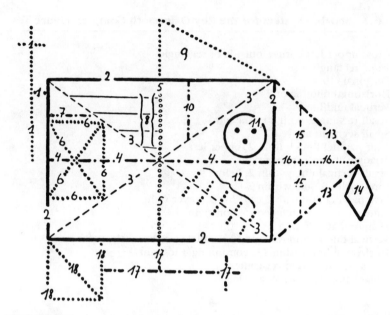

FIGURE 6.3   Scoring units for the Rey-Osterrieth Complex Figures Test.
From Osterrieth, P.A. (1944). Le test de copie d'une figure complex. *Archives de Psychologie, 30,* 233. Reprinted by permission.

maze has its own set of norms that give the percentage of control subjects who passed it. The test has been reported to be sensitive to right hemisphere dysfunction (Fenton, Elithorn, Fogel, & Kerr, 1963) and left hemisphere damage (Colonna & Faglioni, 1966). Although this test has not been widely used in clinical settings, the results of the research conducted to date suggest that it may be a useful screening device.

TABLE 6.3   Percentile Norms for Accuracy Scores on the Rey-Osterrieth Figure

	Percentile			
Trial	25	50	75	100
Copy	31	32	34	36
Memory	18	22	27	35

Source: Lezak, M.D. (1976). *Neuropsychological assessment.* New York: Oxford University Press. Copyright © 1976, Oxford University Press. Adapted by permission.

Block Design and Other Construction Tests

Block design tests require the patient to reproduce a pattern, usually using multicolored blocks. The most frequently used block test is a part of the Wechsler Intelligence Scales, the Block Design subtest. In this task, the patient is presented with a picture of a red-and-white design that must be constructed using either four or nine red-and-white blocks. The blocks have been designed such that each block has two sides that are completely white; two sides that are completely red; and two sides that are half red and half white, split along the diagonal. McFie (1975) has shown that this test is most sensitive to right hemisphere lesions. Additionally, it has been shown that performance on the test will be depressed in left hemisphere injuries, especially those with severe involvement of the varietal lobe of the brain (McFie, 1960). Golden (1977c) demonstrated that the test is effective in identifying over 80% of patients with either right hemisphere or diffuse dysfunction.

The Wechsler Scales Block Design Test was based on the Kohs Blocks test. The two tests differ in that in the Kohs Blocks Test each block is four-colored—red, white, blue, and yellow (Goldstein & Scheerer, 1953). The designs used also differ, and many of them are far more difficult than those employed by the Wechsler version of the test; however, administration and basic interpretation are essentially the same. Although the widespread use of the Wechsler Block Design Test has made administration of the Kohs Block Test redundant in most cases, the Kohs Block Test may be useful in bringing out mild visuoconstructive deficits in very bright individuals.

An alternative to block design tests is the Stick Construction Test (Butters & Barton, 1970). The patient is presented with several roughly 3-inch-long plastic sticks that are ¼-inch square. The patient is then shown designs made with the sticks and asked to replicate them. The task requires both normal and rotated copying. The task is sensitive to postcentral lesions and can provide lateralizing signs (Beaumont & Davidoff, 1992).

Complex visual–spatial functioning also can be assessed using three-dimensional construction tasks. One simple method is to use two subtests from the 1960 Revision of the Stanford-Binet. The Tower and the Bridge (levels II and III, respectively) can be administered simply and easily. The client is simply asked to make a tower (i.e., stack) with a series of 1-inch square blocks and a "bridge" with three blocks. Failure on either of these simple tasks is evidence of serious impairment. Somewhat more frequently used is the Test of Three-Dimensional Block Construction (Benton, Hamsher, Varney, & Spreen, 1983). In this test, the client is presented with 29 loose blocks and with a three-dimensional model ranging from a 6-block pyramid to a 15-block, four-level construction. She is then instructed to use the loose blocks and put some of them together so that they look like the model. For each construction, the time to completion is recorded with an upper limit of 5 minutes per construction. Each model is scored for the number and types of errors in accordance with the test instructions (omissions, additions, substitutions, and displacements). The score can then be compared with reference data available with the test. The test is sensitive to moderate and severe impairment.

Raven's Progressive Matrices

This test was originally designed as a culture-free measure of intelligence (Raven, 1960). Although subsequent research has found that the test did not meet this goal, it does appear to offer a measure of nonverbal reasoning. The test is quite easy to administer and can be given with little formal training. There are no time limits, and the test generally takes from 40 minutes to 1 hour. It consists of 60 items grouped into five series, plus 2 sample items. Each item contains a pattern problem with one part missing and from four to eight pictured inserts, one of which contains the correct pattern (see Figure 6.4). The subject points to the pattern piece he feels will complete the larger

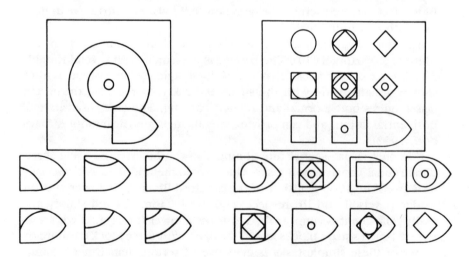

FIGURE 6.4   Examples of the Raven's Progressive Matrices Test.

pattern. Alternatively, the patient can write the response on an answer sheet. There is also a version for children and adults of low intellectual level—the Coloured Progressive Matrices.

Norms are available from ages 8 to 65. Raw scores are converted to percentiles. Seven percentile levels are given for age groups ranging from 20 to 65. For finer-scaled scoring, Peck (1970) has developed a set of percentiles much more specific than those that accompany the test. The effectiveness of the Progressive Matrices in identifying organically impaired individuals appears related to the extent of the injury (Zimet & Fishman, 1970). Thus, the poorer the performance, the more likely the presence of dysfunction.

Trail Making Test

The Trail Making Test (Army Individual Test, 1944) has been widely used as an easily administered test of visual-conceptual and visuomotor tracking. Like most other tests that have a large attention Al component, it is highly sensitive to the effects of brain injury (Reitan, 1958). It is given in two parts, A and B (see Figure 6.5). The patient is asked to draw lines connecting consecutively numbered circles on one work sheet (Part A), and then is asked to connect the same number of consecutively numbered and lettered circles on another work sheet by alternating between letters and numbers (Part B). The examiner records both the time required and the number of errors made, as well as pointing out the errors to the patient so they can be corrected. The time this takes is reflected in the total time required to complete each section.

As is the case for all test performance scored on speed alone, it must be remembered that *allowances need to be made for normal aging, because psychomotor speed tends to decrease with age*. The Trail Making Test is no exception to this, as performance time has been found to decrease with each succeeding decade (Davies, 1968). Table 6.4 demonstrates this trend in normal control subjects.

In general, cutoff scores are used for determining whether performance is impaired on the Trail Making Test. For younger individuals, aged 20 to 39, normal performance time on Part A should be 50 seconds or less and 79 seconds or less for Part B. The combined time to complete both Parts A and B should be less than 110 seconds. However, when these cutoff criteria are applied to normal individuals in their seventies, the scores misclassify an average of 91% as being brain damaged. Therefore, it is important to account for the age of the patient being tested and for the distributions of scores achieved

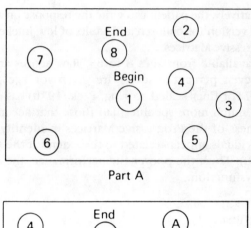

Part A

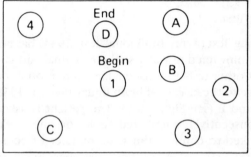

Part B

FIGURE 6.5 Practice samples of the Trail Making Test.

by normal older subjects. The values presented in Table 6.4 may be used in lieu of the standard cutoff scores when testing older patients.

When the time taken to complete Part A is relatively far less than that needed to complete Part B, it is likely that the patient has difficulty in complex conceptual tracking or sequencing. Slow performance at any age on one or both parts of the test points to the likelihood of brain damage, but does not indicate whether the problem is one of motor slowing, uncoordination, visual scanning difficulties, poor motivation, or conceptual confusion (Lezak, 1976).

Clock Drawing

The Clock Drawing Test is a simple, quick clinical screening for visual-spatial and constructional deficits. It has been used as a part of a stan-

TABLE 6.4   Trail Making Test Scores[a] for Normal Control Subjects

Age	20–39 (N = 180)		40–49 (N = 90)		50–59 (N = 90)		60–69 (N = 90)		70–79 (N = 90)	
Part	A	B	A	B	A	B	A	B	A	B
Percentile										
90	21	45	22	49	25	55	29	64	38	79
75	26	55	28	57	29	75	35	89	54	132
50	32	69	34	78	38	98	48	119	80	196
25	42	94	45	100	49	135	67	172	105	292
10	50	129	59	151	67	177	104	282	168	450

[a]Scores are in seconds.

Source: Davies, A. (1968). The influence of age on Trail Making Test performance. *Journal of Clinical Psychology, 24.* Adapted by permission.

dard brief MSE in neurology for some time (e.g., Strub & Black, 1977). The test requires a sheet of paper and a pencil. The patient is told to draw the face of a clock with all the numbers on it and to make it large. Once the patient has completed her drawing, she is told to draw the hands at 20 to 4. The instructions can be repeated or paraphrased as needed, but no other help should be offered.

The task is scored as follows: A 10-point scoring system is used. A score of 10 is awarded if it is a normal drawing with the numbers and hands in roughly the correct positions. The hour hand should be distinctly different from the minute hand and approaching 4 o'clock. A score of 9 is received if there are slight errors in the placement of the hands (not exactly on the 8 and 4, but not on one of the adjoining numbers) or one missing number from the face of the clock. Eight points are given with more noticeable errors in the placement of the hour and minute hand (off by one number), or if the number spacing shows a gap. A score of 7 is given if the hands are placed significantly off the mark (more than one number), or there is inappropriate spacing of the numbers (all numbers on one side of the clock). Six points are scored with inappropriate use of the clock hands (use of a digital display or circling of the numbers despite repeated instructions, or the crowding of numbers at one end of the clock or a reversal of numbers. The patient receives a score of 5 when there is a perseverative or otherwise inappropriate arrangement (e.g., numbers indicated by dots). Also this score is given if the hands are represented but do not clearly point at a number. Four points are received when numbers are absent, written outside of the clock, if they are distorted in sequence, or if the hands are not clearly represented. A score of 3 points is given when numbers and face are no longer connected in the drawing or the hands are not recognizably present. A score of 2 is given when the drawing reveals some evidence that the instructions were understood, but the representation of the clock is vague, at best. Typically there is an inappropriate spatial arrangement of numbers. Finally, a score of 1 point is attained when there is no attempt or the attempt is not recognizable.

Currently available norms suggest that scores of 7 to 10 represent normal functioning (Sunderland et al., 1989; Wolf-Klein, Silverstone, Levy, & Brod, 1989). A score of 6 is thought to be borderline. Scores of 5 or less are rare in normal functioning individuals.

AUDITORY FUNCTIONS

As is the case with vision, the verbal and nonverbal components of auditory perception appear to be functionally distinct (Milner, 1962). Also as with vision, there are many psychological techniques for assessing verbal auditory functions. However, in contrast to visual perception, neuropsychology has paid comparatively little systematic attention to nonverbal auditory functions. Thus although there is a tremendous variety of verbal tests involving audition, the psychological examination of the nonverbal aspects of auditory perception is limited to only a few techniques.

Every comprehensive neuropsychological evaluation provides some opportunity to evaluate the auditory perception of verbal material. This is also the case for a neuropsychological screening. When the examiner presents orally problems of judgment and reasoning, learning and memory, the opportunity also arises to conduct an informal assessment of the patient's auditory acuity and comprehension, as well as of processing capacity. Significant deficits in the perception and comprehension of speech can become readily apparent quite rapidly during the course of administering most psychological tests.

If a few tasks with simple instructions requiring only motoric responses or one or two word answers are given, however, subtle problems with auditory processing may be missed. These include difficulty in processing or retaining lengthy messages, although responses to single words or phrases may be accurate; inability to handle spoken numbers without a concomitant impairment in processing other forms of speech; or an inability to process information at high levels in the auditory system when the ability to repeat them accurately remains intact. In the absence of a primary hearing disorder, any impairment in the individual's capacity to recognize or effectively process speech typically indicates a lesion in the dominant cerebral hemisphere (Milner, 1962).

When impairment in auditory processing is suspected, the clinician can couple an auditorily presented test with a similar task presented visually. This enables the clinician to compare the functioning of both perceptual systems under similar conditions. If the patient demonstrates a consistent tendency to perform better under one of the two conditions, the possibility of neurological impairment of the less efficient perceptual system exists. Pairs of tests can be readily found or developed for most verbal tests at most levels of difficulty. For instance, a series of tasks requiring both written and mental computations can be used.

Nonverbal Auditory Perception

As the vast majority of a person's behavior is organized around verbal signals, the potential for overlooking nonverbal auditory functions is present. The recognition, discrimination, and comprehension of non-symbolic sound patterns, such as music, tapping patterns, rhythms, and meaningful noises (sirens, automobile horns, thunder, etc.), are subject to impairment as much as is the perception of language sounds. Dysfunction in nonverbal auditory perception tends to be associated with brain damage in the right temporal region (Milner, 1962).

Another important area that should be at least screened involves what are referred to as *paralinguistic* behaviors in communication. It has been estimated that 93% of what people communicate in interactions with others occurs through nonverbal means. These include vocal quality, loudness, speech intelligibility, fluency (ease of production), and prosody (Hartley, 1990). Prosody refers to patterns of intonation (pitch), rhythm (rate), and stress (loudness) in utterances, all of which carry a good deal of information about the speaker, such as emotional status and certain personality features. Features the astute clinician can be looking for include recognizing the intended meaning of nonliteral forms of speech, such as metaphors, proverbs, jokes, or indirect requests; making inferences from stories heard; appreciating and producing affective elements of communication; and producing coherent and socially appropriate conversation (Hartley, 1990).

Seashore Rhythm Test

Most assessment devices for nonverbal auditory functioning use sound recordings. The Seashore Rhythm Test (Seashore, Lewis, & Saetveit,

1960) is probably the most widely used test since it was incorporated into the test battery developed by Halstead (1947). This test requires that the patient listen to pairs of tone groups and determine whether the tone groups in the pair are the same or different from one another. The test is scored in terms of the number of errors. Normal individuals tend to make fewer than five or six errors; a greater number of errors suggests dysfunction. Because a component of the test assesses ability to attend and make rapid decisions, the tape should not be stopped once it has started, and the patient should be encouraged to keep up with the tape.

The examiner can also improvise tests for nonverbal auditory perception. The original Halstead and Wepman Aphasia Screening Test requires the patient to identify a tune ("America") the examiner either whistles or hums. Alternatively, the examiner can ask the patient to identify any popular melody, such as "Happy Birthday" or "Home on the Range." An adult raised in the United States who is unable to recognize any popular melody is typically demonstrating an amusia that suggests right temporal lobe damage. The examiner can also assess pitch perception with a pitch pipe, asking the patient to report which of two sounds is higher. (These sounds can also be hummed or whistled.) Recognition of rhythmic patterns can be evaluated by requiring the patient either to discriminate similar and different sets of rhythmic taps or to mimic patterns tapped out by the examiner with a pen or pencil on the table top. The addition of a memory component increases the sensitivity of these tasks to perceptual impairment. Memory techniques, however, should be added only if the individual being assessed demonstrates adequate memory in other modalities.

An alternative to the preceding test is the use of the Rhythm Scale of the Luria-Nebraska Neuropsychological Battery (Golden, Hammeke, & Purisch, 1985). This scale has all of the components mentioned previously, and many of the stimuli used are on tape so that each patient receives the same stimuli in the same manner. One added feature of this scale is that normative data are available for comparison. One drawback to using the Rhythm Scale is that the clinician must purchase the complete Luria-Nebraska Battery, which, while not as costly as some other comprehensive neuropsychological assessment test batteries, requires a substantial investment.

When the perceptual task is as simple as asking for a discrimination between three evenly spaced taps and three taps spaced so that the first two are close together with a lag between the second and third taps, more than one failure suggests defective nonverbal auditory perception. The patient who fails two or three of as many as five attempts on this type of discrimination task should be given an additional five trials with similar material to clarify whether she misunderstood the instructions or was having difficulty concentrating on the task—or whether a perceptual deficit indeed exists. The pairing of similar tasks involving both verbal and nonverbal material can help clarify the interpretation of the patient's difficulties.

TACTILE FUNCTIONS

Assessments of defects of touch perception have employed a variety of different techniques to elicit or measure the different ways in which tactile perception can be disturbed. Most of the techniques present simple recognition or discrimination problems. A few involve more complex behavior.

Tactile Recognition and Discrimination Tests

The detailed examination for finger agnosia (Kinsbourne & Warrington, 1962) includes three tactile tests that require no elaborate equipment. The patient is asked to close his eyes (alternatively, the patient can be blindfolded) and place the hands, palms down, on the working surface for all of these tests. These tests should be given first with the patient's eyes open to assure that the tasks are understood. In the *In-between Test*, the examiner touches two fingers simultaneously, having instructed the patient to tell the number of fingers in between the two that are touched. The *Two Point Finger Test* requires that the examiner touch two places on the same or different fingers; the patient is asked to tell whether one or two fingers were touched. In the *Match Box Test*, the examiner slips a small match box between two of the patient's fingers or touches the sides of two different fingers with two match boxes. The patient is required to tell which fingers were touched. *Of these three tests, the In-Between Test has consistently been found to be the most clinically useful* (Lezak, 1976). Patients with finger agnosia consistently had difficulty differentiating their fingers or relating one to another. Control subjects with some form of cortical dysfunction but no evidence of finger agnosia performed these tests without error.

If the clinician decides to use the approach used by Benton et al. (1983), then the test consists of 60 items broken into 3 sections: (1) with the hand visible, localization of single fingers touched by the examiner with the pointed end of a pencil (10 trials on each hand); (2) with the hand hidden from view, localization of single fingers touched by the examiner (10 trials on each hand); (3) with the hand hidden from view, localization of fingers touched simultaneously by the examiner (10 trials on each hand). The mode of response is left to the patient. She can name the touched fingers, point to them on an outline drawing of the stimulated hand, or call out their numbers. Throughout the test, the patient's hands rest on the table with the palm up, and fingers extended and separated slightly. In those individuals with a spastic movement disorder in which the hand and fingers cannot be positioned to allow for a valid assessment, finger localization testing is limited to the unaffected hand. Several performance patterns have been reported using this approach (Benton et al., 1983). *Normal performance* is reflected by a score of 51 to 60 (single-hand score of 25 to 30, with right-left difference of 0 to 3 points. *Borderline normal* performance results from a total score of 49 to 51 (one single-hand score of 26 to 27 and one single-hand score of 23 to 24, with right-left difference of 0 to 3 points. *Bilateral symmetric impairment* is present when single-hand scores are less than 26, with right-left differences of 0 to 3 points. Generally, when the right-left score is greater than 4 points, the greatest defect is reflected by the hand with the poorest performance.

Object recognition without the aid of vision (stereognosis) is commonly performed in a standard neurological examination. The patient is asked to close his eyes and is required to recognize by touch common objects such as a coin, pencil, key, and so forth. Each hand is assessed separately. Size and texture discrimination can be easily assessed. *Adults with no evidence of brain injury can perform tactile recognition and discrimination tests with total accuracy. A single error or even evidence of hesitancy is a strong suggestion that this function is impaired.* Such deficits are typically associated with lesions on the contralateral hemisphere (Weinstein, 1964).

Reitan-Klove Sensory Perceptual Examination

This test combines much of the tactile perceptual examination techniques discussed previously into a single package, which is comparatively easy for an experienced clinician to administer. It is important, however, that the clinician receive some training in the administration of this series of tests; they can easily be administered improperly, yielding useless findings. Proper administration is essential for useful and interpretable results.

This test was developed by Reitan and Klove (Reitan, undated) and draws on a long history of similar tests used in neurology. The first part of the test evaluates the presence of sensory suppressions, using double simultaneous stimulation in the tactile, auditory, and visual modalities. Tests for the perception of single stimulation are included, because suppressions cannot be scored unless it is clear that the patient is able to perceive unilateral stimulation. The patient is asked to close her eyes and place her hands on the table. The examiner then proceeds randomly to touch either one of the patient's hands, either side of the patient's face, both hands, both sides of the face, or one hand and the opposite side of the face. *It is important that bilateral stimulation be done simultaneously and with equal pressure or else the patient will be receiving two unilateral stimuli, thus defeating the purpose of the examination.* There should be no discernible pattern to the touching, and each hand as well as each side of the face should receive an equal number of both unilateral and simultaneous stimulations. The test is scored in terms of errors.

To assess the presence of auditory perception deficits, the examiner stands behind the patient and rubs his fingers together slightly behind, but close to, the patient's ears. The clinician then asks the patient to tell on which side the noise was made—right, left, or both at once. The examiner should be careful to make the stimulus noise just audible to the patient and to assess unilateral as well as bilateral simultaneous perceptual functioning. As above, total errors are scored.

Assessment for visual suppression is done in a similar manner. The examiner sits about 3 feet away from the front of the patient and asks the patient to fixate on the examiner's nose. The examiner's hands are then held at about an arm's length away from the examiner's body, and one or two fingers are moved slightly. The patient is then asked on which side the movement occurred—left or right. Bilateral presentations also occur. The examiner again should be sure to give the patient an equal number of unilateral and double simultaneous stimulations. The upper, middle, and lower portions of the patient's visual fields should be assessed in this manner.

If no primary sensory deficit is in evidence, as indicated by correct identification of unilateral stimulations, even one error in double simultaneous stimulation can be indicative of cerebral dysfunction. The clinician must, however, be certain that the suppression error was a valid suppression and not the result of a temporary lapse in the patient's attention. *Genuine suppressions are quite rare but are almost always indicative of brain injury.*

The Sensory-Perceptual Examination also includes a set of tests of more complex tactile perceptual functioning. The *Finger Agnosia Test* identifies the patient's capacity for recognizing which finger is touched while blindfolded (or with eyes closed). For this test, each finger on each hand is touched in random sequence by the examiner, with the patient telling the examiner which finger was touched. Some type of finger identification system that the patient can understand and remember should be devised before the test actually begins. Generally, a simple numbering system, with the thumb being finger number one and the little finger being number five, works well. (The reader is directed to the previous section for more detailed instructions.) Similarly, the Fingertip Number Writing Test examines the blindfolded patient's ability to recognize numbers written on the fingertips. It is important that the examiner make certain that the patient knows the alphabet and how the selected numbers are to be drawn. The patient first practices with eyes open. The average adult may make two or three errors on each hand. Errors greater than three on either side suggest defective performance. In the absence of an aphasic condition or sensory deficit, a contralateral lesion is suspected when the patient displays an error difference between the two hands. Regardless of the side on which performance was deficient, a tactile perceptual dysfunction is implied by poor performance on this task.

Two tests for astereognosis are also included in the examination. The first is the Coin Recognition Test, where the patient is asked to identify by touch alone a penny, dime, and nickel placed in each hand separately and in both hands at the same time. When both hands are being simultaneously tested, one type of coin is placed in one of the patient's hand while a different coin is placed in the other. The Tactile Form Recognition Test involves the recognition of simple geometric shapes—a circle, square, Greek cross, triangle—by touch. For this test, the patient first places the right hand in a shadow box, and one of the shapes is placed in the hand. The patient is then required to identify, as rapidly as possible, the shape that was placed in the hand by pointing to the correct shape in an array of shapes in front of her. The task is then repeated with the left hand, using the shapes in a different sequence. Both trials are then repeated, each time using a different sequence of shapes. The Tactile Form Recognition Test is scored for both accuracy in shape identification and for total response time for each hand. The normal adult rarely makes any errors, and the response time for each shape is generally less than two seconds. Reitan and Wolfson (1985) offer limited normative performance data.

MANUAL MOTOR FUNCTIONING

It is important to include a measure or measures of manual motor control, speed, and dexterity in a neuropsychological screening battery. All such tests are timed speed tests that either have an apparatus with a counting device or require a countable response from the patient. Such tests have been useful in the detection of lateralized brain dysfunction.

Finger Tapping Test

Probably the most widely used of these tests of motor functioning is the Finger Tapping Test (Reitan & Davison, 1974), which was originally called the Finger Oscillation Test by Halstead (1947). It consists of a tapping key with a device for recording the number of taps. Each hand performs five 10-second trials, with brief rest periods interspersed between trials. The score for each hand is the average across the five trials. Normal right-handed individuals average 50 taps per 10-second trial for their dominant hand and 45 taps for the left hand. As with other motor tasks, age and sex will affect expected performance levels. The presence of cortical damage tends to have a slowing effect on the finger tapping rate. Lateralized lesions may result in a marked slowing of the tapping rate of the hand contralateral to the lesion. However, such effects do not appear with enough frequency or consistency to warrant the use of this test as a screening for lateralized damage. Diffuse damage will lead to a generalized slowing of the tapping rate of both hands. *In general, the clinician can expect to see about a 10 % d reference in the tapping rates of the two hands, with the dominant hand being faster*.

Grip Strength

As we have noted, examining the patient's level of performance and comparing performance on both sides of the body can be useful in determining the integrity of brain functioning. Clinicians have realized that intensity or strength of voluntary motor activity can also be a reliable indicator of brain functions. Many neuropsychologists use some strength-of-grip measure in comprehensive evaluations. A measure of grip strength can also be used in a screening evaluation.

Reitan and Davison (1974) established the hand dynamometer as having clinical value for such purposes. Testing the strength of a patient's grip requires the use of a dynamometer, which can be adjusted to the size of the patient's hands. The patient is asked to extend his preferred hand downward and is then instructed to squeeze as hard as possible. Two trials are given to each hand in alternating fashion. The final score for each hand is the average of the two trials. The dominant hand result should be 10% greater than that of the nondominant hand.

Clinicians who may wish to consider using the Grip Strength Test should be warned that while the test is a reasonably good indicator of brain dysfunction in a number of instances, it cannot be used as the sole measure; it is not accurate enough to do so. Additionally, hand dynamometers are not inexpensive. A recent survey of dynamometer manufacturers and suppliers revealed an average cost of over $230.

The Purdue Pegboard Test

The Purdue Pegboard Test, which was developed as a test of manual dexterity for employment selection procedures, has been found to be neuropsychologically sensitive (Purdue Research Foundation, 1948). The test has also been used in the investigation of lateralized lesions (Costs, Vaughan, Levita, & Farber, 1963) and motor dexterity among brain-damaged patients.

Following standardized instructions, the patient places pegs in holes with his left hand, right hand, and then both hands simultaneously. Each trial lasts for 30 seconds, so that the total actual testing time is only 90 seconds. The score is the number of pegs placed correctly. Average scores of normative groups range from 15 to 19 for the right hand, 14.5 to 18 for the left hand, 12 to 15.5 for both hands, and 43 to 50 for the sum of all three trials. Females tend to be able to place one or two more pegs correctly on each of the trials.

Although brain-injured patients as a group tend to perform more poorly than non–brain-damaged individuals, patients with right hemisphere lesions may be almost completely nonfunctional when using the left hand (see Table 6.5). Cutoff scores developed for the Purdue Peg-

TABLE 6.5   Purdue Pegboard Average Test Scores in Normal and Brain Damaged Populations

	Left-brain– damaged patients	Right-brain– damaged patients	Normal control subjects
Right hand	9	10	14
Left hand	10	0	13

Source: Lezak, M.D. (1976). *Neuropsychological assessment*. New York: Oxford University Press. Copyright © 1976, Oxford University Press. Adapted by permission.

TABLE 6.6   Cut-Off Scores for the Purdue Pegboard Test[a]

	Age < 60	Age 60 +
Preferred hand	< 13	< 10
Nonpreferred hand	< 11	< 10
Both hands	< 10	< 8

[a]Indicates cortical dysfunction

Source: Lezak, M.D. (1976). *Neuropsychological assessment.* New York: Oxford University Press. Copyright © 1976, Oxford University Press. Adapted by permission.

board Test have been proven to be 70% accurate in predicting a lateralized lesion in one study, 60% accurate in predicting lateralization in the cross-validation of the original study, and 89% accurate in identifying brain dysfunction in general for both samples (Costa et al., 1963). Two separate sets of cutoff scores were developed for older and younger patients (Table 6.6). More extensive normative data can be found in a text by Spreen and Strauss (1991). In addition, for patients of all ages, a brain lesion is likely to be present whenever score of the nonpreferred hand exceeds that of the preferred hand, or the score of the preferred hand exceeds that of the nonpreferred hand by three or more points. Slowing on one hand is suggestive of a dysfunction in the contralateral hemisphere, and bilateral slowing typically occurs with diffuse or bilateral brain damage. It is important to note that as a result of performance changes over time, right-left difference scores or ratios tend not to be reliable (Reddon, Bill, Gauk, & Maerz, 1988) and should be avoided.

Because the total testing time, including instructions and practice, rarely exceeds 5 minutes, the Purdue Pegboard can be a highly efficient method of screening for cortical dysfunction and detecting a lateralized lesion. Because it is not only brief, but also unlikely to fatigue a patient unduly, it can be readily included in most neuropsychological test screening batteries; however, the test's size and weight may place limits on its portability in some situations.

7

Screening Tests for Verbal Functions

TESTS FOR APHASIA

Almost any verbal test may be classified as an aphasia test, because patients with language disorders tend to perform more poorly than do patients without such disorders. Specific tests for aphasia, however, differ from other verbal assessment devices in that they focus on disorders of symbol formulation as well as on associated agnosias and apraxias (Benton, 1967). Such tests have been designed to elicit samples of an individual's behavior in each of the various communication/language modalities of listening, speaking, reading, writing, and gesturing. The important issue is the selection of a device that can sample all such language behaviors quickly and efficiently.

While aphasia screening tests are not designed to replace the careful examination of language functions afforded by comprehensive language assessment batteries, they can signal the presence of a disorder and may even call attention to its specific characteristics. But they do not provide the fine discriminations of the more complete aphasia test batteries (Eisensen, 1973). Because these tests do not require technical knowledge of speech pathology for satisfactory administration or interpretation, they can be easily administered and interpreted by clinicians who are not familiar with aphasia syndromes.

Aphasia Screening Test

Since its introduction, this has become the most widely used of all aphasia tests. The Aphasia Screening Test (AST) or one of its many variations has been incorporated into many formally organized neuropsychological test batteries. As originally devised by Halstead and Wepman (1959), the AST has 51 items that cover all the elements of aphasic disabilities as well as the most common language problems. Total administration time rarely exceeds 30 minutes and is frequently much shorter. The AST has no rigid scoring standards. The emphasis of the test is on determining both the presence and, to a lesser extent, the nature of communication problems. Errors are coded into a diagnostic profile that can provide a description of the pattern of a patient's language disabilities. The test is not designed to assess performance on the basis of severity of the problem. However, the more areas of involvement noted and the more a single area is involved, the greater the severity of the dysfunction.

Reitan included the AST with a number of other different tests in the Halstead-Reitan Neuropsychological Test Battery, which is described elsewhere. He reduced the original test to 32 items, but still handled the data in a descriptive fashion in much the same manner as originally intended (Reitan, undated). This shortened version of the AST is the one most commonly used and is readily available. Table 7.1 and Figure 7.1 present the tasks in the AST as well as the organization of the items.

A second revision of the AST appeared in Russell, Neuringer, and Goldstein's (1970) amplification of the Halstead-Reitan Test Battery. This recent version of the original Halstead and Wepman test is called the "Aphasia Examination" and contains 37 items. It is essentially the same as the Reitan revision, except that four easy arithmetic problems and the task of naming a key were added. A simple error counting system was also established for use with a computerized scoring and diagnostic classification system. As Lezak (1976) notes, the scoring system and derived six-point rating scale indicate the severity of an aphasic disorder, but not its nature.

Finally, a very short version of the AST has been developed, consisting of four tasks (Heimburger & Reitan, 1961). The tasks are:

1. Copy a square, Greek cross, and triangle without lifting the pencil from the paper.
2. Name each copied figure.
3. Spell each name.
4. Repeat: "He shouted the warning"; then explain and write it.

TABLE 7.1   Modified Halstead-Wepman Aphasia Screening Test Items

Task	Instructions to patient
1. Copy SQUARE (A)	FIRST, DRAW THIS ON YOUR PAPER. (point to square, item A). I WANT YOU TO DO IT WITHOUT LIFTING YOUR PENCIL FROM THE PAPER. TRY TO MAKE IT ABOUT THE SAME SIZE (elaborate as necessary). If patient is concerned about making a heavy or double line, note that only a reproduction of the shape is necessary. If patient encounters difficulty in shape reproduction, encourage patient to do his or her best. If the task is not accomplished reasonably well on the first attempt, ask patient to try again.
2. Name SQUARE	WHAT IS THAT SHAPE CALLED?
3. Spell SQUARE	WOULD YOU SPELL THAT WORD FOR ME?
4. Copy CROSS (B)	DRAW THIS ON YOUR PAPER (point to cross). GO AROUND THE OUTSIDE LIKE THIS UNTIL YOU GET BACK WHERE YOU STARTED (examiner draws a finger line around the edge of the figure). MAKE IT ABOUT THE SAME SIZE. Additional instructions are given in the same manner as those used for the square as needed.
5. Name CROSS	WHAT IS THAT SHAPE CALLED?
6. Spell CROSS	WOULD YOU SPELL THAT WORD FOR ME?
7. Copy TRIANGLE (C)	Similar to instructions for 1 and 4.
8. Name TRIANGLE	WHAT IS THAT SHAPE CALLED?
9. Spell TRIANGLE	WOULD YOU SPELL THAT WORD FOR ME?
10. Name BABY (D)	WHAT IS THIS? (show item D).
11. Write CLOCK (E)	NOW I AM GOING TO SHOW YOU ANOTHER PICTURE BUT DO NOT TELL ME THE NAME OF IT. DON'T SAY ANYTHING OUT LOUD. JUST WRITE THE NAME OF THE PICTURE ON THE PAPER (show item E).
12. Name FORK (F)	WHAT IS THIS? (show item F).
13. Read 7 SIX 2 (G)	I WANT YOU TO READ THIS (show item G). If patient has difficulty, attempt to determine if any of the stimulus figure can be read.
14. Read M G W (H)	READ THIS (show item H).
15. Reading I (I)	READ THIS (show item I).
16. Reading II 0)	TRY TO READ THIS (show item J).
17. Repeat TRIANGLE	NOW I AM GOING TO SAY SOME WORDS. I WANT YOU TO LISTEN CAREFULLY AND SAY THEM AS CAREFULLY AS YOU CAN. SAY THIS WORD: TRIANGLE.
18. Repeat MASSACHUSETTS	THE NEXT ONE IS A LITTLE HARDER BUT TRY TO DO YOUR BEST. SAY: MASSACHUSETTS.

TABLE 7.1 (*Continued*)

Task	Instructions to patient
19. Repeat METHODIST EPISCOPAL	NOW REPEAT THIS ONE: METHODIST EPIS-COPAL
20. Write SQUARE (K)	DON'T SAY THIS WORD OUT LOUD (point to item K). JUST WRITE IT ON YOUR PAPER. If the patient prints the word, ask him or her to write it in script or cursive.
21. Read SEVEN (L)	READ THIS WORD OUT LOUD (show item L).
22. Repeat SEVEN	NOW, I WANT YOU TO SAY THIS AFTER ME: SEVEN.
23. Repeat and explain HE SHOUTED THE WARNING	I AM GOING TO SAY SOMETHING THAT I WANT YOU TO SAY AFTER ME. LISTEN CAREFULLY: HE SHOUTED THE WARNING. NOW YOU SAY IT. PLEASE EXPLAIN WHAT THAT SENTENCE MEANS. Sometimes the examiner will have to ask for additional explanations by asking the kind of situation to which the sentence refers. The patient must indicate that danger is impending.
24. Write HE SHOUTED THE WARNING.	NOW, WRITE THAT SENTENCE ON THE PA-PER. The sentence can be repeated if necessary.
25. Compute 85 − 27 = (M)	HERE IS AN ARITHMETIC PROBLEM. COPY IT ON THE PAPER AND TRY TO SOLVE IT (show item M).
26. Compute 17 x 3 =	NOW DO THIS ONE IN YOUR HEAD. HOW MUCH IS 17 × 3?
27. Name KEY (N)	WHAT IS THIS? (show item N).
28. Demonstrate use of KEY	SHOW ME HOW TO USE THIS IF YOU HAD ONE IN YOUR HAND (show item N).
29. Draw KEY (N)	NOW, PLEASE DRAW A PICTURE THAT LOOKS LIKE THIS ONE. TRY TO MAKE YOUR KEY LOOK ENOUGH LIKE THE ONE IN THE PICTURE SO THAT SOMEONE WOULD KNOW IT WAS THE SAME KEY AS IN THE DRAWING (point to item N).
30. Read (O)	WOULD YOU READ THIS? (show item O).
31. Place LEFT HAND TO RIGHT EAR	PLEASE DO WHAT IT SAID?
32. Place LEFT HAND TO LEFT ELBOW	NOW, I WANT YOU TO PUT YOUR LEFT HAND ON YOUR LEFT ELBOW. The patient should realize that this is not possible.

Source: Boll, T.J. (1981). The Halstead-Reitan Neuropsychological Battery. In S.B Filskov & T.J. Boll (Eds.), *Handbook of clinical neuropsychology*. New York: Wiley-Interscience. Copyright © 1981. Reprinted by permission of John Wiley & Sons, Inc.

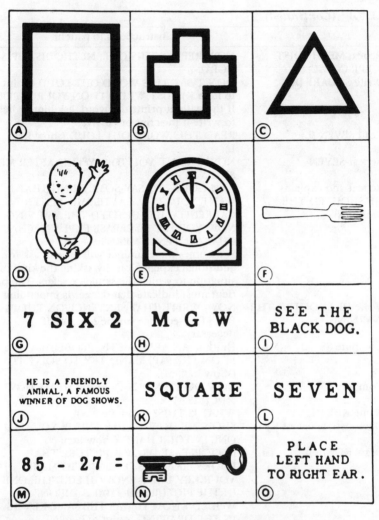

FIGURE 7.1 Stimulus figures for testing cerebral functions.
From Boll, T.J. (1981). The Halstead-Reitan Neuropsychological Battery. In S.B. Filskov & T.J. Boll (Eds.), *Handbook of clinical neuropsychology*, p. 593. New York: Wiley-Interscience. Copyright © 1981. Reprinted by permission of John Wiley & Sons, Inc.

This overly shortened version of the test can help in discriminating between individuals with left and right hemisphere lesions. It is generally expected that individuals with right hemisphere lesions would have difficulty in performing the drawing tasks well and that patients with left-hemisphere damage would be unable to perform the verbally based tasks without some difficulty.

The Token Test

The Token Test is very easy to administer, easy to score, and, for almost anyone who has completed grade 4, easy to perform with few if any errors (Boller & Vignolo, 1966; DeRenzi & Vignolo, 1962). It is remarkably sensitive to disrupted linguistic processes that are central to aphasic disorders, even when the patient's basic ability to communicate has remained intact. The test also can identify those brain-damaged individuals whose other disabilities may be hiding or masking a concomitant aphasic disorder, or whose problems with symbol processing are comparatively subtle and not readily observable in most situations.

The Token Test is comprised to 20 "tokens," usually cut from heavy construction paper, thin sheets of plastic, or wood. They come in two shapes—circles and rectangles; two sizes—large and small; and five colors—red, yellow, blue, green, and white. The only requirement that the test makes of the patient is that she understand the token names and the verbs and prepositions in the instructions. Diagnosis of the limited number of individuals whose language problems are so severe as to prevent them from cooperating with the testing is not likely to depend on formal testing. Almost all other patients with brain damage can respond to the simplest level of instructions on the test (Lezak, 1985). There are five sections, totaling 62 instructions, to the test, which increase in complexity from one section to the next with respect to the instructions given to the patient (see Table 7.2 and 7.3).

While the Token Test seems easy to administer, the examiner must be careful not to modify the rate of delivery inadvertently in response to the quality of the patient's performance. Items that are failed on the first section of the test should be repeated and, if performed correctly on the second administration, scored separately from the first response. When the second but not the first administration of an item is performed successfully, only the second administration is counted, under the assumption that a large number of initial errors is likely to result from a number of variables, such as inattention and lack of interest. Each correct response earns one point, so that the highest possible score is 62. When

TABLE 7.2   The Token Test

Part I

(Large rectangles and large circles only are on the table)
1. Touch the red circle.
2. Touch the green rectangle.
3. Touch the red rectangle.
4. Touch the yellow circle.
5. Touch the blue circle.
6. Touch the green circle.
7. Touch the yellow rectangle.
8. Touch the white circle.
9. Touch the blue rectangle.
10. Touch the white rectangle.

Part 2

(Large and small rectangles and circles are on the table)
1. Touch the small yellow circle.
2. Touch the large green circle.
3. Touch the large yellow circle.
4. Touch the large blue rectangle.
5. Touch the small green circle.
6. Touch the large red circle.
7. Touch the large white rectangle.
8. Touch the small blue circle.
9. Touch the small green rectangle.
10. Touch the large blue circle.

Part 3

(Large rectangles and circles only)
1. Touch the yellow circle and red rectangle.
2. Touch the green rectangle and the blue circle.
3. Touch the blue rectangle and yellow rectangle.
4. Touch the white rectangle and the red rectangle.
5. Touch the white circle and the blue circle.
6. Touch the blue rectangle and the white rectangle.
7. Touch the blue rectangle and the white circle.
8. Touch the green rectangle and the blue circle.
9. Touch the red circle and the yellow rectangle.
10. Touch the red rectangle and the white circle.

Part 4

(Large and small rectangles and circles)
1. Touch the small yellow circle and the large green rectangle.
2. Touch the small blue rectangle and the small green circle.
3. Touch the large white rectangle and the large red circle.
4. Touch the large blue rectangle and the large red rectangle.

TABLE 7.2 (*Continued*)

5. Touch the small blue rectangle and the small yellow circle.
6. Touch the small blue circle and the small red circle.
7. Touch the large blue rectangle and the large green rectangle.
8. Touch the large blue circle and the large green circle.
9. Touch the small red rectangle and the small yellow circle.
10. Touch the small white circle and the large red rectangle.

Part 5

(Large rectangles and circles only)
1. Put the red circle on the green rectangle.
2. Put the white rectangle behind the yellow circle.
3. Touch the blue circle with the red rectangle.
4. Touch—with the blue circle—the red rectangle.
5. Touch the blue circle and the red rectangle.
6. Pick up the blue circle or the red rectangle.
7. Put the green rectangle away from the yellow rectangle.
8. Put the white circle before the blue rectangle.
9. If there is a black circle, pick up the red rectangle. (There is no black circle.)
10. Pick up the rectangles, except the yellow one.
11. Touch the white circle without using your right hand.
12. When I touch the green circle, you take the white rectangle. (Wait a few seconds before touching the green circle.)
13. Put the green rectangle beside the red circle.
14. Touch the rectangles, slowly, and the circles, quickly.
15. Put the red circle between the yellow rectangle and the green rectangle.
16. Except for the green one, touch the circles.
17. Pick up the red circle—No, the white rectangle.
18. Instead of the white rectangle, take the yellow circle.
19. Together with the yellow circle, take the blue circle.
20. After picking up the green rectangle, touch the white circle.
21. Put the blue circle under the white rectangle.
22. Before touching the yellow circle, pick up the red rectangle.

Source: Lezak, M.D. (1976). *Neuropsychological assessment.* New York: Oxford University Press. Copyright © 1976, Oxford University Press. Adapted by permission.

scoring, it is important for the examiner to note whether the patient makes the distinction between instructions such as "touch" and "pick-up" as directed in Part 5 of the test.

holler and Vignolo (1966) have slightly modified the original test format. They give the full record of scores achieved by their standardization groups. With an optimal cut-off score, they were able to classify correctly 100% of normal individuals, 90% of patients without language disorders but with right hemisphere lesions, and 65 % of non-

TABLE 7.3   Token Arrangement

Row 1
Large circles in order: red, blue, yellow, white, and green
Row 2
Large squares in order: blue, red, white, green, and yellow
Row 3
Small circles in order: white, blue, yellow, red, and green
Row 4
Small squares in order: yellow, green, red, blue, and white

aphasic patients (Table 7.4). Cross-validation on another sample resulted in significant shrinkage (Hartje, Kerschensteiner, Poeck, & Argass, 1973). Spreen and Strauss (1991) offer a somewhat different version of the Token Test, which has an expanded scoring system. Using this expanded scoring, the test becomes sensitive to even minor impairments of receptive language.

The last section of the Token Test (Part 5), consisting of items involving relational concepts, was found to identify correctly only one fewer patient as aphasic than did the entire 62 item test. This finding suggests that Part 5 of the test could be used without the other 40 questions to identify those patients with left hemisphere dysfunction who have been misclassified as nonaphasic because their deficits in symbol formulation are too subtle to impair their communicative abilities for most ordinary purposes (Lezak, 1983).

Identification of Objects by Use

Another quick test of intact language can be achieved by having the patient identify common objects by their use as a means to identify the

TABLE 7.4   Cut-Off Scores for the Token Test

Partial score	Max. score	Normal/control	Aphasic
Part 1	10	10	9 or less
Part 2	10	9	8 or less
Part 3	10	9	8 or less
Part 4	10	9	8 or less
Part 5	22	18	17 or less
Total test	62	58	57 or less

Source: Lezak, M.D. (1976). *Neuropsychological assessment*. New York: Oxford University Press. Copyright © 1976, Oxford University Press. Adapted by permission.

presence of ideational dyspraxia. This type of task is a common feature found in more extensive language assessment batteries (Eisenson, 1954; Porch, 1971). One study of the incidence of ideational dyspraxia found that 34% of aphasic patients were not able to identify the use of objects, while only 6% of nonaphasic individuals with left hemisphere lesions, and none of the patients with right hemisphere damage, were unable to do so (DeRenzi, Pieczuro, & Vignolo, 1968). These findings suggest that *this technique can be readily used in a rapid screening for language difficulties as long as it is remembered that while failure on such a task greatly increases the probability of an associated aphasic disorder, success does not rule out the presence of language problems.*

VERBAL FLUENCY

A large number of patients experience changes in speed and fluency of verbal production following damage to the brain. *Greatly reduced verbal production often accompanies most forms of aphasia, but it does not necessarily indicate the presence of aphasia.* Impaired verbal fluency is also associated with damage to the frontal regions of the brain, particularly the left frontal region anterior to Broca's area (Benton, 1968; Milner, 1967).

A fluency problem may be manifested in speech, reading, or writing. More often than not, it will affect all three activities. There are a number of techniques for quickly checking verbal fluency in the course of a screening for possible brain dysfunction.

Boston Naming Test

Because there is a high incidence of naming difficulties in language disorders as well as in other neuropathological conditions, most comprehensive language assessments contain a naming task. The Boston Naming Test (Kaplan, Goodglass, & Weintraub, 1983) is a popular 60-item test. It has been designed to offer a detailed examination of naming abilities and is well standardized across ages. There are 60 line drawings ranging from simple high-frequency vocabulary words to highly infrequent words. They are presented one at a time, and two prompting cues can be given if the client does not produce the word spontaneously. Detailed scoring instructions are included in the test manual, and good normative data for both adults and children are available.

TABLE 7.5   Age and Education Adjustments for Controlled Word Association Test

Education	Age 25–54	Age 55–59	Age 60–64
Males			
< 9	+ 14	+ 15	+ 17
9–11	+ 6	+ 7	+ 9
12–15	+ 4	+ 5	+ 7
> 15	+ 0	+ 1	+ 3
Females			
< 9	+ 9	+ 7	+ 12
9–11	+ 6	+ 7	+ 9
12–15	+ 4	+ 5	+ 7
> 15	+ 0	+ 1	+ 3

Source: Lezak M.D. (1976). *Neurological assessment.* New York: Oxford University Press. Copyright © 1976, Oxford University Press. Adapted by permission.

Controlled Word Association Test

The production of spoken words beginning with a designated letter has been studied a great deal by Benton (1973). The associative value of each letter of the alphabet, with the exceptions of *X* and *Z*, was determined in a normative study using control subjects who were not brain injured (Borowski, Benton, & Spreen, 1967). *Control subjects of low ability were found to perform less well than brighter brain-damaged patients. This result highlights the need to account for the patient's premorbid verbal skills when evaluating verbal fluency.*

The Controlled Word Association Test consists of three word naming trials using the letters, *F*, *A*, and *S*, respectively. The examiner asks the patient to say as many words as he can think of that begin with the given letter of the alphabet, excluding proper nouns, numbers, and the same word with a different suffix. The score is the sum of all correct words pronounced in the three one-minute trials, adjusted for age, sex, and education (Table 7.5). The adjusted scores are then converted to percentiles (Table 7.6).

An alternative mode of presentation provides the patient with predetermined sets (Isaacs & Kennie, 1973). The patient is asked to name as many items as she can from four successive categories: colors, animals, fruits, and towns. The patient names items in the first category until 10 item names are given or until no more can be remembered, at which point the next category is announced, and so on. Lezak (1983) notes that healthy elderly individuals were able to recall an average of 31.2

TABLE 7.6   Controlled Word Association Test Percentiles for Adjusted Scores

Adjusted score	Percentile	Adjusted score	Percentile
54–62	95 +	36	40–44
52–53	90–94	35	40–44
49–50	85–89	34	35–39
46–48	80–84	33	30–34
44–45	75–79	31–32	25–29
43	70–74	29–30	20–24
41–42	65–69	27–28	15–19
40	60–64	25–26	10–14
38–39	55–59	24	5–9
37	50–54	< 23	< 4

Source: Lezak, M.D. (1976). *Neuropsychological assessment*. New York: Oxford University Press. Copyright © 1976, Oxford University Press. Adapted by permission.

names overall, while brain-damaged individuals were able to recall only 15 or less.

WRITING FLUENCY

Word Fluency

A written test for word fluency first appeared in the Primary Mental Abilities Test (Thurstone, 1958; Thurstone & Thurstone, 1962). The patient is required to write as many words beginning with the letter *S* as possible in 5 minutes. Next the patient is asked to write as many four-letter words beginning with C as he can in 4 minutes. The average individual can produce 65 words within the 9-minute total writing period (Lezak, 1983). Milner (1967) found that the performance of individuals with left frontal lobectomies was significantly impaired on this test when compared with patients whose surgery was confined to the right hemisphere.

READING FLUENCY

The Stroop Test

The Stroop Test (Stroop, 1935) can be used as a measure of verbal fluency as well as a general test of cognitive efficiency. The materials for the Stroop include three white cards, each of which contains 10 rows of five items. Randomized color names—blue, green, and red—are in black

TABLE 7.7   Normal Subject Performance on the Stroop Test

		Trial[a] 1	Trial[a] 2	Trial[a] 3
50–item[b]	Mean	24.7	32.9	40.9
cards	SD	8.7	12.6	8.1
100–item[c]	Mean	45.6	47.2	68.3
cards	SD	9.1	10.3	14.5

[a]Trial 1 = Read black print.
 Trial 2 = Read color print.
 Trial 3 = Name color dots.
[b]Talland (1965).
[c]Nehemkis and Lewinsohn (1972).

print on the first card (A). Card two (B) is identical to the first, except that each color name is printed in some color other than the one it names. Card C displays colored dots in the same array of three colors. There are three trials, each consisting of a different task. On the first trial, the patient reads Card A. During trial two, the patient is asked to read the names of the colors on card B; for trial three, she is asked to name the color of the print on card C. Throughout the three trials, the patient is instructed to read or name colors as fast as possible. Table 7.7 presents some normative performance data for the Stroop.

Golden (1978) developed another version of the Stroop Test that has been demonstrated to be useful in the identification of brain damage. This version consists of three 8 1/2-by-11-inch pages. Each item on the first page is one of the following words: red, green, or blue. These words are repeated on the page in a largely random order. The second page consists of 100 items, as does page one, but each item is the sequence XXXX. On this page, each XXXX is printed in red, green, or blue ink. The third page consists of the words printed on page one printed in the colors used on page two; however, a word and the color in which it is printed do not match. Therefore, "red" can be printed in either blue or green ink, "green" in red or blue ink, and "blue" in red or green ink.

The instructions for page I require that the patient read down each column as quickly as possible, pronouncing the words printed. For page 2, the basic instructions remain the same, except that the patient is told to name the color of the XXXX. Finally, on the third page, the patient is instructed to name the color of the ink rather than the word itself. Fortyfive seconds are allotted for each page. The score is the number of items correctly finished within the time limit on each page. These scores are then converted into standardized T-scores using tables in the test manual.

This version of the Stroop was found to differentiate reliably between normal, psychiatric, and brain-damaged patients. On page 2, normal patients were able to complete 70 to 90 items, psychiatric patients completed 60 to 80 items, and brain-damaged individuals were able to complete less than 60 on average (Golden, 1976). Golden (1979) notes that this version of the Stroop can be used to localize lesions: good performance on pages I and 2 in conjunction with poor performance on page 3 is characteristic of frontal lobe dysfunction, especially on the left side. Patients with damage to the right hemisphere tend to perform normally on page I but poorly on pages 2 and 3. Left hemisphere damage that is not located in the frontal regions tends to lead to poor performance on all pages of the test.

The Stroop has also been found to be useful in the identification of dyslexia. Equivalent scores on pages 2 and 3 are never seen in literate adults (Golden, 1979). Thus, if the page-3 score is within 10% of the page 2 score, there is a high possibility of dyslexia, as this implies that the normal interference problem (words interfering with color naming) has not occurred and that there is a lack of word-reading responses.

Recent research has indicated that the Golden (1978) version of the Stroop Test may be differentially sensitive to HIV-related cognitive slowing (Martin et al., 1992). In this version, a computerized version of the Stroop recorded the reaction time of those taking the test. Although these are still preliminary in nature, this technique may prove to be a highly useful administration in the near future.

ACADEMIC SKILLS

As this edition is being prepared, the Wide Range Achievement Test 3 (WRAT3; Wilkinson, 1993) has just been announced for release. The advance materials for the test indicate that the test features a new national stratified sample, new grade ratings, scaling and item analysis, as well as newly designed test forms and new absolute scales. Two equivalent forms of the test also have been developed that will allow the clinician to perform pretesting and posttesting. In addition, the WRAT3 will offer the capability for performing a profile analysis for assessing strengths or weaknesses, and comparing or combining the results of the equivalent forms. These changes offer much promise and increased utility for this widely used device. No information has yet been provided concerning changes in the time required for administration; however, it is anticipated that the administration time will be largely unchanged.

Lezak (1983) notes that few neuropsychological batteries or screening tests contain measures of academic skills such as reading, writing, or arithmetic. However, impairment in these areas can have profound implications on a patient's vocational competence and ultimate adjustment. The inclusion of such measures, therefore, is an important consideration for any screening of neuropsychological functioning. There are a variety of easily and quickly administered academic skills assessment devices available, such as the Wide Range Achievement Test–Revised (Jastak & Wilkinson, 1984) and Peabody Individual Achievement Tests (Dunn & Markwardt, 1970; Markwardt, 1989). Sections of each of these tests canoe used to assess accurately some aspects of reading fluency.

Lezak (1983) supports the use of a more comprehensive reading test such as the Gates-MacGinitie Reading Tests (Gates & MacGinitie, 1969). These are paper and pencil multiple-choice tests in four primary levels as well as three grade and high school levels. The highest level, Survey F. contains norms for grades, 10, 11, and 12. The highest level of this form (last quarter of grade 12) is the best to be used with adults, although the ceiling may be too low for college graduates.

The Gates-MacGinitie tests measure different aspects of reading separately. The first subtest, Speed and Accuracy, has a 4-minute limit and determines how rapidly the patient reads with comprehension. The second subtest, Vocabulary, involves simple word recognition, while the last subtest measures ability to understand written passages (Comprehension). Both Vocabulary and Comprehension scores tend to be lower when verbal fluency is impaired. If verbal fluency is essentially intact but the higher level conceptual and organization functions are impaired, a marked difference between Vocabulary and Comprehension, with Vocabulary higher, will be seen.

Tests similar to the Gates-MacGinitie are the Woodcock Tests of Reading Mastery (Woodcock, 1973). This series of tests includes sections on letter identification, word recognition, word attack (use of phonetic skills), word comprehension, and passage comprehension. Subtests can be used either together or independently, depending on the specific problem area being addressed.

A welcome addition to the psychologist's armamentum of tests of academic achievement is the Wechsler Individual Achievement Test (WIAT, 1992). Although the test is actually designed for individuals ranging in age from 5 to 19 years, it has uses with an adult population as well. Specific subtests of the WIAT include Basic Reading—designed to assess the ability to decode letters and words; Mathematics Reasoning—a measure of the ability to reason mathematically; Spelling—a subtest that measures the ability to encode dictated sounds and words; Reading Comprehension—designed to assess reading comprehension via reading of a printed passage and responding to an orally presented question; Numerical Operations—a multiset subtest that examines the ability to write dictated numerals, the ability to solve computation problems involving various operations, and the ability to solve simple algebraic equations; Listen Comprehension—an assessment of understanding of orally presented words; Oral Expression—a task that requires the individual to express a target word orally as well as describe a scene, give directions, and explain steps; and Written Expression—a task in which the individual is asked to write on a topic described in the test material. All subtests have extensive standardized instructions for administration and scoring. Excellent normative data are provided in the comprehensive testing manual. If a patient's score is below what would be expected normatively given the patient's age and education, then a potential deficit in the area of poor performance exists that may reflect significant cognitive dysfunction. Interpretively, the WIAT's normative data can be used in a manner similar to the way a PIAT-R or WRAT-R would be used when a patient's age is greater than that of the reference population. A full administration can take up to 60 minutes. The clinician, therefore, may wish to pick and choose carefully the subtests he or she feels are needed to provide the requisite information for the screening procedure.

8

Screening for Memory Functions

A disruption of memory functioning is a common complaint that accompanies a wide variety of clinical conditions and, as such, has many potential causes. Memory is not a unitary construct. Therefore, a screening of memory functioning should cover the span of immediate memory, the addition of new information to recent memory, the extent of recent memory, and the capacity of the individual for new learning (Lezak, 1983). Ideally, these different memory functions would be systematically reviewed through the major input and output modalities with both recall and retrieval techniques. However, in those cases where memory problems do not seem to be primary in nature, thoroughness can be sacrificed for a number of practical considerations such as time, patient cooperation, and fatigue.

With most adults, the WAIS-R is a generally good starting point. It directly enables the examiner to assess the span of immediate memory as well as the extent of remote memory (via the Information subtest) stored in verbal form. The longer Arithmetic and Comprehension subtest questions also offer the clinician indirect information on the duration and stability of the immediate verbal memory trace. The MSE (described in detail in chapter 5) can augment information gathered from the patient with a delayed verbal memory task requiring the patient to recall three of four spoken items after five minutes of intervening material, as well as with questions to assess the retention of ongoing experience at the minimal level necessary for independent living. The addition of an immediate memory and retention task, using simple designs, and a test of learning ability will offer a more complete review of the major dimensions and modalities of memory.

When performance on these tasks is not significantly depressed relative to the patient's best performance on other tasks, and particularly when performance on tests of remote memory is not significantly better than the handling of learning tasks, the clinician can make the assumption that memory and learning are reasonably intact. Pronounced deficits on the general review of memory may suggest the need for a more in-depth memory assessment, which involves the systematic comparison between functions, modalities, and the length, type, and complexity of content. This can be done by the clinician doing the screening if she has had the appropriate training and time is available, or it may point up the need for the patient to be referred out for a comprehensive evaluation of cognitive functions.

A relatively poor performance only on tests of immediate memory and learning may indicate that the patient is severely depressed and may point up the need for such a differential determination. Impaired immediate memory and learning are also common early symptoms of a variety of neurological conditions that can ultimately result in general cognitive deterioration. As the still relatively intact patient with neurological dysfunction experiences his failing abilities, he may also be appropriately depressed, a situation that can further compound the differential diagnostic picture. It must be remembered, however, that depressed patients typically are unlikely to demonstrate cognitive deficits other than memory loss and psychomotor slowing or retardation. In contrast, a patient with an abnormal neurological status will likely show additional defects in processing, and a comprehensive evaluation will likely be necessary to detail the nature and extent of the dysfunction.

VERBAL MEMORY AND LEARNING PROBLEMS

There are a large number of techniques that can be used to screen for verbal memory and learning problems. The almost unlimited possibilities for combining different kinds of verbal stimuli with input and output modalities and presentation formats have resulted in an explosion of verbal memory tests. Many of them were developed in response to specific clinical problems or research questions. Only a few have received enough use or sufficiently careful standardization to have reliable norms. Moreover, because of the lack of systematic comparisons between different verbal memory tests, their relative utility and potential interchangeability are actually unknown. For this reason, our discussion of specific assessment tools will be limited to those few tests and standardized batteries that have been demonstrated to be useful to the clinician.

The clinician's choice of memory screening tests depends on clinical judgment rather than on scientific demonstration that any given test is most suitable for answering a specific question. Even with the many tests available, the examiner may occasionally find that none will suit the needs of a specific patient and may be required to devise his own individual memory test for screening purposes. The experiences clinician also may wish to use portions of existing batteries to address specific types of memory difficulty.

Digit Span

The Digit Span subtest of the WAIS-R (Wechsler, 1981) is the most widely used test of verbal immediate memory. The test has two general sections, both consisting of seven pairs of random sequences of numbers. In the Digits Forward segment, the examiner reads aloud number sequences that are from three to nine digits long, and the patient must repeat each segment exactly as it is heard. The Digits Backward portion of the subtest operates in much the same fashion, the major difference being that the patient must say the digits read by the examiner in reverse order. Each section of Digit Span discontinues when the patient fails to repeat both number sequences of a pair of equal length.

This test produces three scores: Digits Forward, Digits Backward, and total Digit Span. The Forward and Backward scores are the number of digits in the longest correctly repeated sequence for each section. The total Digit Span score is the sum of the scores of the two sections. All but a few elderly individuals are able to recall at least four digits forward and three backward, but fewer than 1% get the maximum nine forward and eight backward. The average adult will be able to recall six digits forward and five backward.

In addition to immediate auditory-verbal memory, Digit Span involves auditory attention. The Digits Backward segment of the test measures not only immediate memory, but also the capacity of the patient to juggle information mentally. The ability to reverse sequences effectively requires both memory and the reversing operation to operate simultaneously, a kind of mental "double tracking" (Lezak, 1976). That Digits Forward and Digits Backward do not involve identical operations is apparent in the score discrepancy of three or more points between the Forward and Backward segments that tends to occur in brain-damaged patients with concentration problems. This is not a common response pattern of brain-damaged individuals who do not have difficulties with concentration and is rarely seen in non–brain-damaged persons (Costa, 1975).

The immediate memory assessed by the Digit Span test tends to be more vulnerable to left hemisphere dysfunction than to either right-sided or diffuse injury. This vulnerability is reflected in factorial studies of brain-damaged and elderly individuals in which, contrary to the results of factor analytic studies of normal groups, a verbal factor contributes significantly to the test performance, whereas the prominence of a memory factor is reduced but not nullified. Additionally, contrary to clinical speculation, anxiety and distractibility do not appear to play as large a role in performance on such tests as once was thought (Guertin, Ladd, Frank, Rabin, & Hiester, 1966).

Because of its memory and attention components, Digit Span remains one of the WAIS-R subtests most sensitive to the effects of any kind of brain injury. *As a general rule, a difference of three or more points between Digits Forward and Digits Backward reflects a concentration deficit of organic origin, and any Digits Forward score office or less in a middle-aged or younger person is suggestive of impaired immediate memory.* Digit Span scores tend to be the lowest immediately following brain injury and generally increase over time, although scores may remain low in relation to other subscale scores even several years postinjury (Wheeler & Reitan, 1963).

Nonsense Syllable Learning

Nonsense syllables have been a popular medium for assessing memory since 1885, when Ebbinghouse first reported on their utility in exploring retention and forgetting. They may be the stimulus of choice when the clinician wants to assess verbal functions while minimizing or controlling the confounding effects of meaning. Noble (1961) has created a useful table of 2, 100 nonsense syllables of the consonant-vowel-consonant (CVC) type, along with their measured associations and meaningfulness values, for use in test syllable sets.

The Nonsense Syllable Learning Test (Newcombe, 1969) is a straightforward recall test with considerable clinical utility. Eight CVC syllables printed on a card in a vertical list are shown to the patient for three minutes, the card is removed, and the patient writes down as many of the syllables as can be remembered. Next there is a 5-minute period in which some nonrelated activity is performed, after which time the examiner, without warning the patient, asks the patient to name the syllables. On both the immediate and delayed recall portions of this test, patients with left-hemisphere damage display poorer performance than patients with right-hemisphere damage.

Rey Auditory-Verbal Learning Test

The Rey Auditory Verbal Learning Test (RAVLT) is a brief, easily administered, paper-and-pencil task that assesses immediate memory span, new learning, susceptibility to interference, and recognition memory. The original version was developed by Rey (1964) and was later adapted by Lezak (1976, 1983) for use with English-speaking individuals.

The test starts as a test of immediate word memory span. For the first trial (of six), the examiner reads a list of 15 words at the rate of I per second (see Table 8.1). Before beginning the list, the patient is told that he will be read a word list and then be asked to repeat as many as he can remember, in any order, when the examiner stops. The examiner writes down the words recalled by the patient in the order recalled. In this way, the patient's pattern of recall can be tracked, noting whether the patient proceeds in a systematic manner, whether he associates two or

TABLE 8.1 Rey Auditory-Verbal Learning Test Words

List A	List B	List C
drum	desk	book
curtain	ranger	flower
bell	bird	train
coffee	shoe	rug
school	stove	meadow
parent	mountain	harp
moon	glasses	salt
garden	towel	finger
hat	cloud	apple
farmer	boat	chimney
nose	lamb	button
turkey	gun	key
color	pencil	dog
house	church	glass
river	fish	rattle

Source: Lezak M.D. (1976). *Neuropsychological assessment.* New York: Oxford University Press. Copyright © 1976, Oxford University Press. Adapted by permission.

three words, or whether his recall is a hit or miss proposition. If the patient asks the examiner whether a word has already been said, the patient should be told; however, this information should not be volunteered, because it may distract the patient and interfere with performance.

When the patient indicates that no additional words can be recalled, the examiner gives a second set of instructions and then rereads the list. The second set of instructions tells the patient that the same list will be read again and that, when it is completed, the patient is to say back as many words as can be remembered. The patient is also asked to repeat the words said the first time and told that the order is not important. The second set of instructions must emphasize the inclusion of the previously said words so that the patient does not think that the test is one of elimination.

The list is reread for trials 111, IV, and V, using the second trial instructions each time. Praise may be given as words are recalled, and the patient may be told the number of words recalled, especially if the patient is able to use the information for reassurance or as a challenge. On the completion of the last trial, the second word list is read, with instructions similar to those for the first word list. Following the reading of the second-list trial, the patient is asked to recall as many words from the first list as he can (trial VI). Should either the first- or second-list presentations be spoiled by interruptions, improper administration, confusion, or premature response on the patient's part, the third word list is available. Following a 20-minute delay, which should be filled with other activities, the patient is then asked to recall as many words from the first list (list A) as he can. Once the delayed recall task is complete, the examiner then asks the patient to identify from printed lists (recognition) as many words as he can from both lists A and B.

The score for each trial is the number of words correctly recalled. A total score, the sum of trials one through five, can also be calculated. Words that are repeated can be noted, as can words that were not on the list (errors or confabulations). Norms for trials one through five are available (Table 8.2) and are broken down by social class and age. Table 8.3 shows the recognition-trial normative data gathered on these groups. Extended normative data are now available for ages 16 to 70 + (Geffen et al., 1990).

Tables 8.4 and 8.5 show the RAVLT scores by age for men and women.

Selective Reminding Test

The Selective Reminding Test (SRT) was first described as a specific procedure to measure verbal lessening and memory during a multiple-trial

TABLE 8.2   Recall for Each Trial of the Rey Auditory-Verbal Learning Test

Group	Trial 1		Trial 2		Trial 3		Trial 4		Trial 5	
	M	SD	M	SD	M	SD	M	SD	M	SD
Manual laborers	7.0	2.1	10.5	1.9	12.9	1.6	13.4	2.0	13.9	1.2
Professionals	8.6	1.5	11.8	2.0	13.4	1.4	13.8	1.1	14.0	1.0
Students	8.9	1.9	12.7	1.7	12.8	1.5	13.5	1.3	14.5	0.7
Elderly laborers[a]	3.7	1.4	6.6	1.4	8.4	2.4	8.7	2.3	9.5	2.2
Elderly professionals[a]	4.0	2.9	7.2	2.9	8.5	2.5	10.0	3.3	10.9	2.9

[a]Ages 70–90 years.

Source: Lezak, M.D. (1976). *Neuropsychological assessment*. New York: Oxford University Press. Copyright © 1976, Oxford University Press. Adapted by permission.

learning task by Buschke (1973; Buschke & Fuld, 1974). Although there is no commercial source for this test, it is highly effective in assessing memory functioning (Spreen & Strauss, 1990). The stimulus material consists of a list of words, index cards containing the first two to three letters of each word on the list, and index cards containing the multiple-choice recognition items. The procedure requires that the examiner read the patient a list of words and that the patient recall as many of these words as possible. Each subsequent learning trial involves the selective presentation of only those items not recalled on the immediately preceding trial. The SRT distinguishes between short- and long-term components of memory by measuring recall items that were not presented on any give trial. The learning rate of patients can also be assessed. Several different versions of the test have been developed (e.g., Hannay, 1986; Hannay & Levin, 1985) including a children's version.

The total test administration time for the test is about 25 to 30 minutes for adults and 10 minutes for children. Scoring the test is somewhat

TABLE 8.3   Recognition Trial for the Rey Auditory-Verbal Learning Test

Manual laborers		Professionals		Students		Elderly laborers[a]		Elderly professionals[a]	
M	SD	M	SD	M	SD	M	SD	M	SD
14.5	0.8	14.9	0.2	14.8	0.3	11.9	1.8	13.6	1.3

[a]Ages 70–90 years.

Source: Lezak, M.D. (1976). *Neuropsychological assessment*. New York: Oxford University Press. Copyright © 1976, Oxford University Press. Adapted by permission.

TABLE 8.4 RAVLT Scores by Age for Men

Trial	(N)	Age groups (years)						
		16–19 (13)	20–29 (10)	30–39 (10)	40–49 (11)	50–59 (11)	60–69 (10)	70+ (10)
	M (SD)							
1—List A		6.9 (1.8)	8.4 (1.2)	6.0 (1.8)	6.4 (1.8)	6.5 (2.0)	4.9 (1.1)	3.6 (0.8)
2		9.7 (1.7)	10.8 (1.9)	8.0 (2.4)	9.0 (2.3)	8.6 (2.0)	6.4 (1.2)	5.7 (1.7)
3		11.5 (1.2)	11.3 (1.6)	9.7 (2.7)	9.8 (2.0)	10.1 (1.6)	8.0 (2.6)	6.8 (1.6)
4		12.8 (1.5)	12.2 (1.8)	10.9 (2.8)	11.5 (1.9)	10.7 (1.9)	8.5 (2.7)	8.3 (2.7)
5		12.5 (1.3)	12.2 (2.2)	11.4 (2.6)	10.9 (2.0)	11.8 (2.6)	8.9 (2.0)	8.2 (2.5)
Total		53.2 (5.4)	54.9 (7.0)	46.0 (10.9)	47.5 (8.3)	47.6 (8.5)	36.7 (8.4)	32.6 (8.3)
Distractor (List B)		6.9 (1.9)	6.5 (1.8)	5.3 (1.6)	6.1 (2.1)	5.0 (2.3)	4.9 (1.6)	3.5 (1.3)
6 (List A retention)		11.2 (1.6)	11.1 (1.7)	9.7 (2.3)	9.7 (2.5)	9.6 (2.9)	7.2 (2.87)	6.4 (1.7)
7 (List A delayed recall)		11.3 (1.7)	10.6 (2.4)	10.4 (2.3)	10.5 (2.7)	10.0 (2.6)	7.1 (3.8)	5.6 (2.6)
Recognition A		14.4 (0.9)	14.2 (0.8)	13.5 (1.5)	14.2 (1.0)	13.9 (0.9)	12.4 (2.8)	11.5 (2.6)
Recognition B		8.4 (2.8)	8.2 (2.7)	4.4 (2.0)	6.9 (2.6)	4.7 (2.9)	4.9 (2.7)	3.0 (2.7)

Source: Geffen, G., Hoar, K.J., O'Hanlon, A.P., Clark, C.R., & Geffen, L.B. (1990). Performance measures of 16– to 86-year-old males and females on the Auditory Verbal Learning Test. *Clinical Neuropsychologist*, *4*, 50. Adapted by permission.

TABLE 8.5 RAVLT Scores by Age for Women

		Age groups (years)						
Trial	M (SD)	16–19 (13)	20–29 (10)	30–39 (10)	40–49 (11)	50–59 (11)	60–69 (10)	70+ (10)
1—List A		7.8 (1.9)	7.7 (1.0)	8.0 (2.0)	6.8 (1.5)	6.4 (1.5)	6.0 (2.2)	5.6 (1.4)
2		10.5 (2.0)	10.5 (2.0)	10.8 (2.1)	9.4 (1.5)	8.2 (2.4)	9.0 (2.0)	6.9 (2.1)
3		12.3 (1.2)	12.2 (2.3)	11.5 (1.7)	11.4 (1.7)	10.2 (2.1)	10.8 (2.0)	8.9 (1.9)
4		12.5 (1.7)	12.0 (1.6)	12.9 (1.3)	11.7 (2.1)	11.1 (1.9)	11.3 (1.4)	10.1 (1.9)
5		13.3 (1.5)	12.9 (1.5)	12.7 (1.3)	12.8 (1.4)	11.6 (2.1)	11.9 (1.6)	10.1 (1.2)
Total		56.5 (6.0)	55.3 (6.6)	55.9 (6.3)	52.1 (7.1)	47.6 (7.7)	49.0 (7.1)	41.6 (6.6)
Distractor (List B)		7.7 (1.3)	7.9 (2.0)	6.5 (1.5)	5.2 (1.3)	4.6 (1.9)	5.3 (1.1)	4.2 (1.9)
6 (List A retention)		11.9 (2.5)	11.6 (2.5)	12.1 (1.9)	11.1 (2.4)	9.9 (2.8)	9.8 (1.6)	7.8 (1.8)
7 (List A delayed recall)		11.4 (2.5)	11.0 (2.0)	12.2 (2.5)	11.1 (2.3)	10.2 (2.7)	10.3 (2.3)	8.3 (2.1)
Recognition A		13.8 (2.0)	14.4 (0.8)	14.2 (1.7)	14.4 (0.8)	13.7 (1.1)	13.8 (1.1)	13.6 (2.0)
Recognition B		7.8 (3.1)	8.0 (2.9)	8.9 (4.1)	7.4 (2.8)	5.7 (2.4)	7.5 (3.6)	7.5 (3.7)

Source: Geffen, G., Hoar, K.J., O'Hanlon, A.P. Clark, C.R., & Geffen, L.B. (1990). Performance measures of 16– to 86–year-old males and females on the Auditory Verbal Learning Test. *Clinical Neuropsychologist, 4,* 51. Adapted by permission.

more complex than average and may take the new user a bit of practice to feel comfortable. If a word is recalled on two consecutive trials, it is assumed to have entered long-term storage (LTS) on the first trial. Once a word enters LTS, it is thought to be in permanent storage and is recorded as LTS on all subsequent trials regardless of the patient's subsequent recall. When a word in LTS is recalled, it is scored as a long-term retrieval (LTR). When a word in LTS is consistently recalled on all subsequent trials, it also is scored as consistent long-term retrieval (CLTR) or list learning on the first of the uninterrupted successful recall trials. Inconsistent LTR refers to recall of a word in LTS followed by subsequent failure to recall the word. It is scored as random long-term retrieval (RLTR). Short-term recall (STR) refers to recall of a word that has not entered LTS. The total recall (Sum Recall) on each trial is the sum of STR and LTR. The number of reminders given by the examiner before the next recall attempt is equal to 12 (Sum Recall of the previous trial). Record by number the order of the patient's recall on each trial (see Figure 8.1). Intrusions of words not on the list also are recorded for each trial. (As noted, the scoring is complex but practice does make it easier.) Full scoring instructions, word lists, and other information are available in the publications referred to earlier.

VISUAL MEMORY FUNCTIONING

Most nonverbal memory tests involve visual memory. In order to test recall without resorting to verbalization, these tests must include a practice response, usually drawing. This, of course, can serve to confound the interpretation of deficient performance, because the patient's failure may arise from a practice deficit, from impaired visual or spatial memory, or from an interaction between these (or other) dysfunctions. Even on recognition tasks that do not call for a practice response, such perceptual defects as visual-spatial inattention may compound assessment of memory difficulties. Therefore the clinician must pay close attention to the quality of nonverbal memory test performance in order to estimate the relative contributions of memory, perceptual, and practice components to the end result of the patient's performance.

To minimize the possibility of verbal mediation, most visual recall test stimuli consist of designs or nonsense figures. However, unless they are quite complex or unfamiliar, geometric designs do not fully control for verbal mediation. Additionally, it is virtually impossible to design a large series of nonsense figures that do not elicit verbal associations.

Name: _____ Date: _____ Patient #: _____
Examiner: _____

Trial	1	2	3	4	5	6	7	8	9	10	11	12	CR	MC	30
throw															
flower															
film															
waver															
soft															
beet															
stream															
helmet															
smoke															
hoed															
blank															
ton															
Reminders															
Intrusions															

Trial 1

Total Recall	_____	(Number words recalled over 12 trials)
LTR	_____	(Words recalled 2x in a row, assumed to be in LTS from this point on)
		Underline word with red, counting blanks. Compute over 12 trials)
STR	_____	(Words not underlined. Compute over 12 trials.)
CLTR	_____	(Words not continuously recalled. Mark with highlighter. Sum over 12 trials.)
RLTR	_____	(Words that are underlined by NOT CLTR. Do not count blanks. Sum over 12 trials.)
Reminders	_____	(Compute over 12 trials. Max.= 144)
Intrusions	_____	(Sum over 12 trials.)
Cued Recall	_____	(Max .= 11)
Multiple Choice	_____	(Max= 12)
30 Minute Recall	_____	(Max. = 12)

FIGURE 8.1 Buschke Selective Reminding Test Record Form.

150

Recognition Tests—The Recurring Figures Test

In the Recurring Figures Test, the stimulus materials consist of 20 cards on which are drawn geometric or irregular nonsense figures (Kimura, 1963). After looking at each of the cards in succession, the patient is shown a pack of 140 cards, one at a time for 3 seconds each. This pack contains 7 sets of 8 of the original 20 designs interspersed throughout the remaining 84 unique cards not previously seen by the patient. The patient must indicate whether a given card already has been seen. A perfect score for the test is 56. False positive responses by the patient are subtracted from the total correct response in order to correct for guessing. In Kimura's original study, the control subjects obtained a mean score of 38.9 when the correction for guessing was figured in. Although there was essentially no difference between the corrected scores for patients with either right or left hemisphere damage, the patients with right hemisphere brain damage had more than twice as many false positives than did the group with left-hemisphere damage. The members of both groups were able to recall geometric shapes much better than the nonsense figures, and the group of patients with left hemisphere damage remembered a much larger proportion of the nonsense figures than was remembered by the group with right hemisphere damage.

In a much shorter variant of Kimura's original test, the stimulus set consists of 8 meaningless figures interspersed with 12 other nonsense figures in three 20-card sets. Identical instructions are used, as is the same scoring system, including the correction for guessing (DeRenzi, 1968). The maximum possible score is 24. Patients with right hemisphere damage demonstrated much poorer performance, obtaining a mean score of 0.13 compared to a mean score of 6.4 obtained by a group with left hemisphere damage.

Tactile Memory—The Tactual Performance Test (TPT)

This test uses the Sequin-Goddard Formboard, which, while originally a visuopractic task, was converted by Halstead (1947) into a tactile memory test by administering it to blindfolded subjects and adding a drawing recall segment to the test. Reitan incorporated this version of the test into his testing battery. Three trials are given in Halstead's administration. Each of the first two trials is done with each hand used singly, with the preferred hand being used first. The third trial uses both hands. The score for each trial is the time to completion (getting all the blocks into the proper holes while blindfolded) in seconds. On completion of the formboard trials, and after the board and the blocks have been removed

TABLE 8.6   Tactual Performance Test Cutoff Scores (Normative Data)

	Total time (min)	Memory	Location
Average performance of normal controls	10.7	6.2	5.9
Cutoff score	15.6	6.0	5.0

Source: Halstead, W.C. (1947). *Brain and intelligence.* Chicago: University of Chicago Press. Adapted by permission.

from the patient's view, the blindfold is removed from the patient. The patient is then given a blank sheet of paper and a pencil and instructed to draw from memory as much of the board as is remembered and to indicate the different shapes and their locations relative to one another on the board. Two scores are obtained from the drawing. The memory score is a simple count of the number of shapes reproduced with reasonable accuracy (e.g., a star without the correct number of points still receives credit as long as the basic star shape is preserved). The location score is the total number of blocks placed in proper position relative to the other shapes and the board.

The cutoff scores developed by Halstead were retained by Reitan for predicting the likelihood of organic impairment (Table 8.6). If the individual being assessed is over 40 years of age, allowances in the cutoff scores must be made. For example, Lezak (1983) notes that a normal group of older subjects averaged a time score of roughly 18 minutes.

Although markedly slowed or defective performance on the TPT or memory trials is associated with brain damage, the nature of the organic dysfunction is not clear. Some investigators have found that patients with right hemisphere injury perform more poorly than do patients with left hemisphere injury (Reitan, 1964). However, opposite results on the recall task, with left brain-damaged patients doing worse, have also been reported (DeRenzi, 1968). Reitan (1964) considers the test to be especially sensitive to frontal lobe dysfunction.

Time differences between trials also offer important information. The difference between the time taken with the preferred hand and that taken with the nonpreferred hand may provide a clue as to the side of the lesion. There is an implicit assumption that learning will occur; thus there should be a steady decrease in the time needed to complete the test from trial one with the preferred hand to trial three with both hands. If trial one takes 7 or more minutes and trial two is in the 3- to 5-minute range, the possibility of a dominant hemisphere lesion exists.

Conversely, if trial two takes as long as trial one or even longer, a nondominant hemisphere lesion must be considered.

MEMORY TEST BATTERIES

The Wechsler Memory Scale

To provide a thorough coverage of the varieties of memory disorders, several batteries of memory tests have been developed. Of all the memory test batteries that have been developed, only the Wechsler Memory Scale (WMS) (Wechsler, 1945) has had more than haphazard normative data supporting its utility until recently. With the addition of the Randt Memory Test (Randt & Brown, 1983), the revised version of the WMS (Wechsler, 1987), and the Memory Assessment Scales (MAS) (Williams, 1991), there are now several such assessment devices. It must be cautioned that even these somewhat more carefully designed and normed tests have normative bases that are limited in their applicability for comparison with the general population. Thus, although the batteries contain useful tests and provide practical guidelines for the conduct of a memory examination, *their norms should be used judiciously and should not be used as unequivocal statements of performance criteria for the tests.*

The WMS contains seven subtests. The first two consist of questions commonly found in a MSE. Subtest I, Personal and Current Information, asks for the patient's age and date of birth, as well as identification of current and recent public officials, both national and local. Subtest II, Orientation, has questions about time and place, including the patient's current location. The third subtest, Mental Control, tests automatism (automatic responses, such as the alphabet) and simple conceptual tracking or sequencing (e.g., counting by 4's from 1 to 67).

The fourth subtest, Logical Memory, tests immediate recall of verbal ideas from two paragraphs that are read to the patient. This form of test assesses immediate free recall following auditory presentation. The first paragraph read to the patient contains 24 memory units or "ideas," and the second paragraph contains 22 units. The patient is given one point for each "idea" that is recalled, with the total score being the number of ideas recalled for each paragraph. Young adults (20- to 29-years-old) average about 9 per paragraph; older adults retain a bit less (about 8 ideas per paragraph). The number of correct ideas retained continues to drop slightly across the adult lifespan until the ages of 80-89 when the average is 6.8 (Hulicka, 1966).

The fifth subtest, Digit Span, is similar to the WAIS Digit Span subtest, but differs in that the WMS version omits the three-digit trial of Digits Forward and the two-digit trial of Digits Backward, and credit is not given for performances of nine forward or eight backward. The scoring is the same as for the WAIS version, where the maximum number of digits recalled, both forward and backward, are summed to yield the total Digit Span.

The sixth subtest is an immediate visual memory drawing task (Visual Reproduction). There are four designs, each of which is shown to the patient for 10-seconds, after which she draws the design from memory as completely as possible. Such tests are particularly sensitive to right hemisphere damage. McFie (1960) found a significant number of impaired design reproductions associated with right hemisphere lesions regardless of the specific site of the lesion. This deficit was not found, however, in patients with left hemisphere damage.

The seventh and last subtest, Associate Learning, tests verbal retention. This task consists of ten word pairs, six forming "easy," that is, meaningful, associations (e.g., read-book) and four "hard" word pairs that are not readily associated (e.g., glass-flower). The list is read a total of three times, with a memory trial following each reading. The total score is one-half the sum of all correct associations to the hard pairs made within five seconds after the stimulus word is read. The highest possible score, therefore, is 21. The standardization group aged 20 to 29 averaged about 8 to 9 on the easy pairs and about 7 on the hard pairs. The standardization group aged 40 to 49 showed little difference on the easy pairs, averaging 8.26, but did less well on the hard association pairs, where they averaged 5.7 word pairs. *After the age of 40, scores on this subtest tend to decline steadily.* Generally, patients with left hemisphere injury tend to do less well on this type of task than do patients with right hemisphere lesions. Total administrative time is 20 to 25 minutes.

The Wechsler Memory Scale's normative population is relatively small (approximately 200) and is composed of an unreported number of age groups between the ages of 25 and 50. No information is given about the intellectual ability of the normative subjects, and its restricted age range stops at that point where the greatest normal changes in memory functioning begin to occur and where the incidence of central nervous system abnormalities increases (Lezak, 1983). Hulicka (1966) has attempted to remedy these deficiencies by reporting normative data which span a greater age range.

Russell (1975) has reported a modified scoring system for the WMS that incorporates retesting of logical memory and visual reproduction approximately 30 minutes after initial assessment. This modification permits six scores to be generated: verbal short-term, verbal long-term, verbal percentage retained, figural short-term, figural long-term, and figural percentage retained. Predictably, patients with left hemisphere damage perform more poorly on the verbal memory tasks, while patients with right hemisphere lesions have more difficulty with the figural tasks.

The WMS has two forms (I and II). It has been found that the forms are not interchangeable (Schultz, Keesler, Friedenberg, & Sciara, 1984). Form II is reportedly a little easier than Form I (Ivison, 1988); however, the difference between the forms can be reduced somewhat by changing the scoring procedures as suggested by Ivison (1988). In those cases in which the examiner wishes to investigate memory functioning over a brief period and is contemplating using the alternative forms of the WMS, this becomes an important issue for consideration.

Wechsler Memory Scale-Revised

An updated, revised, and expanded version of the WMS was introduced in 1987, the Wechsler Memory Scale-Revised (WMS-R) (Wechsler, 1987). Among the significant changes to the test were the inclusion of much better normative data that is stratified at nine age levels, replacement of the single Memory Quotient with five memory composite scores, the addition of new subtests assessing figural and spatial memory as well as a delayed recall feature, and the revision of scoring procedure for several of the subtests to improve the accuracy of the scoring.

The first subtest, *Information and Orientation*, covers simple biographical data, orientation, and common information such as "Who is the president of the United States?" *Mental Control*, designed to assess overlearned information, is unchanged from the original version of the test; however, the scoring has been revised to eliminate extra credit for fast performance. *Figural Memory*, a new subtest, requires the patient to view a set of abstract designs and then identify the designs seen when shown a larger set of designs. The next section, *Logical Memory*, is comparable with that section of the original WMS, but story A has been revised slightly to eliminate dated references. A new story has been substituted for the original story B. Scoring changes have made the rules more exhaustive and objective. *Visual Paired Associates I* is a newly developed subtest designed to look at visual learning. The patient is asked to learn the color associated with each of six abstract line drawings. Up to six trials are provided to learn the pairs. *Verbal Paired Associates I* is similar to the original WMS "Associate Learning"; however, the revised version has eight word pairs (four easy and four difficult) rather than the 10 pairs in the WMS. *Visual Reproduction I* is a slightly revised version of the WMS subtest. In this subtest, the patient is required to draw from memory simple geometrical designs that each are exposed for 10 seconds. The revised version has four designs, two of which are new. Scoring rules have been expanded and made more specific. The *Digit Span* subtest is largely the same with the change that both the forward and backward series begin with items that are shorter by one digit. A new subtest, *Visual Memory Span*, is a visual-spatial analogue of the Digit Span test. On this task, the patient is asked to touch a series of colored squares in a predetermined order, which is first demonstrated by the clinician. The remaining four subtests, *Logical Memory II*, *Visual Paired Associates II*, *Verbal Paired Associates II*, and *Visual Reproduction II*, are the delayed recall trials of the immediate memory subtests. They are started 30 minutes after the first presentation of stories. As the test has increased somewhat in length and complexity, the administration time has also increased to roughly 45 minutes.

The initial validity data presented in the test manual was very good. Some expected shrinkage was seen in the cross-validation research. As was the case with the original WMS, the WMS-R is still primarily a test of verbal learning (Bornstein & Chelune, 1988; Chelune & Bornstein, 1988; Loring, 1990). In addition, when calculating the indices (General, Verbal, Visual), verbal memory performance continues to contribute more heavily (Spreen & Strauss, 1991). Despite these potential limitations, the WMS-R is still a highly useful device and should be considered for use in any assessment of memory functioning in a variety of populations (Gold, Randolph, Carpenter, Goldberg, & Weinberger, 1992; Roth, Conboy, Reeder, & Boll, 1990).

Memory Assessment Scales

To date, the newest complete memory battery is the MAS (Williams, 1991). The MAS was developed to assess verbal and nonverbal attention, concentration, and short-term memory; verbal and nonverbal learning and immediate memory; and memory for verbal and nonverbal material following a delay interval. Measures of recognition, intrusions during verbal learning recall, and retrieval strategies are also provided. The device was designed to be usable at bedside, is portable, and has straightforward scoring procedures with easily calculated scores.

The MAS consists of 12 subtests based on seven memory tasks. Subtest one, *List Learning*, is an auditory verbal learning task requiring the client to recall a list of 12 common words, three of each from four semantic categories (countries, colors, birds, and cities). Up to six trials for learning can be presented. The examiner also can assess intrusions as well as the success of clustering strategies allowing for an analysis of the underlying processes affecting performance. *Prose Memory* is an auditory verbal prose recall task similar to WMS logical memory subtests. The client is asked to recall a short story from memory and is asked 9 questions about the story. This subtest also acts as an interference task for the next subtest. *List Recall*, the next subtest, requires the client to recall the words presented in the List Learning subtest. The patient is asked to recall words within semantic categories as well as perform a recognition trial by selecting the learned words from a printed list of 24 alternatives. Additional scores for intrusions, success of clustering, and list recognition can be calculated and analyzed. *Verbal Span* is a standard digit span-type of task. *Visual Span* is a nonverbal analogue of the Verbal Span subtest. In this test, an array of randomly distributed stars is placed before the patient, and the patient must reproduce a specific sequential pattern presented by the examiner. *Visual Recognition* assesses recognition memory for geometrical designs. The patient is shown a design, presented with a distracter task, and then asked if the design next presented is the same or different from the originally presented design (items 1 to 5). For the remainder of the subtest (items 6 to 10), the patient is asked to select the design seen from an array of designs. In the next section, *Visual Reproduction*, the client is required to reproduce a geometrical design displayed for a brief time. There also is a distracter task presented between design presentation and reproduction. The drawings are scored for presence or absence of specific details. *The Names-Faces* subtest is an association learning task. The client is required to learn the names of individuals who are portrayed in photographs. Following learning trials, the client is presented with photographs and is asked to recognize the correct name from a brief list of alternatives. The last four sections involve delayed recall. In the *Delayed List Recall* subtest, the patient is asked to free recall the words presented in the List Learning section and then recall the words within semantic categories as prompted by the examiner. *Delayed Prose Recall* requires the patient to recall the story from memory and then he is asked nine questions concerning details of the story. For *Delayed Visual Recognition*, the client is presented with 20 geometrical designs, 10 of which were those presented in the immediate learning trial. Finally, the

Delayed Names-Faces Recall subtest requires the client to recognize the names of individuals presented earlier in the Names-Faces subtest.

The MAS requires roughly 30 to 45 minutes for administration and has been standardized for use with individuals ranging in age from 18 to 90 years. Scoring is simple and straightforward. Scores can be plotted on a subtest profile that is on the front of the response booklet (see Figure 8.2). Information is provided concerning total intrusions, clustering effectiveness, cuing, and recognition. Excellent normative data are provided and matched according to U.S. census data, as well as by age decade and education.

Overall, the MAS is an excellent addition to the clinician's testing repertoire; however, it must be noted that appropriate time be devoted to learning the administration of the MAS and the clinician cannot expect to be able to validly administer the test right "out of the box." Used carefully and appropriately, the MAS can provide a wealth of information regarding a client's memory functioning.

Rivermead Behavioural Memory Test

The Rivermead Behavioural Memory Test (RMBT) (Wilson, Cockburn, & Baddeley, 1985) differs from most other published tests of memory in its direct attempt to sample memory functioning that is characteristic of everyday life rather than the traditional doctor's office learning and memory tasks typified by the WMS-R and MAS. The battery consists of seven basic subtests including (1) remembering a name (given the photograph of a face); (2) remembering a personal item (which is hidden and the patient must remember to ask for at the end of the test; (3) recall of a message after a delay; (4) common object recognition (the patient is shown 10 photographs and must recognize them out of a set of 20 alternatives shown after a delay period; (5) facial recognition (five faces to be selected from a set of 10 alternatives after presentation of the 5 photographs); (6) a task where the patient is required to remember a route around the testing room; and (7) recall of a short prose passage, both immediately after presentation and after a delay.

Complete instructions are in the test manual. The tests are administered in a fixed order, and total administration time is about 25 minutes. The overall test is scored in one of two ways. The first method generates a "screening score" by scoring a task either as a 1 (for an adequate response) or 0 (for partial or complete failure). The average unimpaired individual should receive a near-perfect score, whereas a score of 3 or

MAS
MAS Record Form

Name _____ Test Date ____ / ____ / ____

Sex _____ Age _____ Education _____ Occupation _____

Handedness _____ Examiner _____

Subtest Profile

Columns (diagonal labels): Verbal Span, Visual Span, List Acquisition, List Recall, Delayed List Recall, Immediate Prose Recall, Delayed Prose Recall, Immediate Names–Faces, Delayed Names–Faces, Visual Reproduction, Immediate Visual Recognition, Delayed Visual Recognition

	Ⓐ	Ⓑ	Ⓒ	Ⓓ	Ⓔ	Ⓕ	Ⓖ	Ⓗ	Ⓘ	Ⓙ	Ⓚ	Ⓛ
Raw score												
Scale score												

Scale Score axis: 19, 18, 17, 16, 15, 14, 13, 12, 11, 10, 9, 8, 7, 6, 5, 4, 3, 2, 1

(right axis: 19, 18, 17, 16, 15, 14, 13, 12, 11, 10, 9, 8, 7, 6, 5, 4, 3, 2, 1)

Normative Table

Verbal Process Scores

	Raw score	Within expectations	Significant
Total Intrusions	____	____	____ (High)
List Clustering			
Acquisition	____	____	____ (Low)
Recall	____	____	____ (Low)
Delayed Recall	____	____	____ (Low)
Cued List Recall			
Recall	____	____	____ (Low)
Delayed Recall	____	____	____ (Low)
List Recognition	____	____	____ (Low)

Summary Scales

	Scale score		Standard score
I) Verbal Span	____		
II) Visual Span	____	Short–term Memory	☐
Total I + II	____		
III) List Recall	____		
IV) Immediate Prose Recall	____	Verbal Memory	☐
Total III + IV	____		
V) Visual Reproduction	____		
VI) Immediate Visual Recognition	____	Visual Memory	☐
Total V + VI	____		
Total III + IV + V + VI	____	Global Memory Scale	☐

FIGURE 8.2 Memory Assessment Scales Record Form cover page.
Copyright © 1991 by Psychological Assessment Resources, Inc. Reprinted by permission.

more failures indicates deficient performance. A more complete profile scoring provides weighted raw scores. Limited normative data are provided in the test materials. Although additional normative data need to be collected, the RBMT is notable for its attempt to provide a somewhat more meaningful and ecologically valid assessment of memory.

9

Screening Tests for Higher Cognitive Functions

In marked contrast to language disorders, dysfunction of higher cognitive processes is not necessarily associated with damage to a specific cortical region. Rather, higher cognitive abilities tend to be generally sensitive to the effects of brain injury regardless of the site of the damage. In actual fact, this is not all that surprising, because cognitive abilities always involve at least (1) an intact system for organizing perceptual information even though specific perceptual abilities may be impaired; (2) an extensive and readily available data base of remembered learned material; (3) the integrity of cortical and subcortical interconnections and interaction patterns that underlie what we commonly refer to as "thought"; and (4) the capacity to process two or more mental events at a time. Additionally, the translation of cognitive activity into overt behavior requires a response modality sufficiently integrated with central activity to transform conceptual experience into manifest behavior and a well-functioning response feedback system for continual monitoring and modulation of output.

Perhaps the most common indicator of cognitive impairment is concrete thinking. The patient may have difficulty forming concepts, categorizing, generalizing from a single instance, or applying procedural rules and general principles. Loss of the abstract attitude frequently results in a preference for obvious, superficial solutions. The patient with organic impairment may not be aware of subtle underlying or intrinsic aspects of a problem and may, therefore, be unable to distinguish the relevant from the irrelevant, the essential from the unessential, or the appropriate from the outlandish. To the extent that the impaired individual is not able to conceptualize abstractly, he must deal with each event encountered as if it were novel, i.e., an isolated experience that requires a unique set of rules.

Cognitive rigidity often occurs in association with concrete thinking. It may be demonstrated as stimulus-bound behavior in which the patient cannot dissociate his responses or pull attention away from whatever is in the perceptual field. It can also appear as the inability to shift perceptual organization, train of thought, or ongoing behavior to meet the changing needs of the environment at any given moment. The cognitively rigid person may seem stuck in one track, unable to switch frame of reference. The stimulus-bound, conceptually inflexible individual is generally unable to plan ahead, initiate activity, think creatively, or adapt to the demands of changing conditions.

Conceptual concreteness and cognitive rigidity are sometimes treated as different aspects of the same dysfunction. When they occur together, they tend to be mutually reinforcing in their effects (Lezak, 1983). Although both are associated with extensive or diffuse injury, significant conceptual inflexibility can be present without the inability to form and apply abstract concepts, particularly when there is damage to the frontal lobes (Zangwill, 1966). Additionally, concreteness does not imply impairment of specific reasoning abilities. Thinking may be concrete even if the patient is able to perform such specific reasoning tasks as making practical judgments. Conversely, when the patient has specific reasoning disabilities, thinking is likely to be concrete (Lezak, 1976).

It is important to recognize that defects in higher-order cognitive functioning are exhibited by a wide range of individuals. For example, psychotic patients with thought disorders, as well as some individuals with limited education, may exhibit conceptual concreteness. Although some psychotic individuals will exhibit cognitive rigidity, it is rare for a nonorganically impaired person to show stimulus-bound behavior. Interpretation of the results of these tests should always be done in the context of a complete history.

Most tests for assessing higher cognitive processes have been designed to look for concrete thinking in one or another form, usually testing concept formation alone or in conjunction with the ability to shift cognitive set (flexibility). Tests of other cognitive processes, such as planning and organization or problem solving and reasoning, do not treat concrete thinking as the primary examination object, but they frequently offer information about it.

TESTS OF CONCEPT FORMATION

Tests of concept formation differ from most other neuropsychological tests in that they focus on the quality or process of thinking more than on the content of the response. A number of these tests have no correct answer per se. Scoring is done through qualitative judgments of the extent to which the response was abstract or concrete, complex or simple. Tests with right and wrong answers might belong in the category of tests of abstract conceptualization to the extent that they yield information about how the patient thinks.

Patients with moderate to severe brain damage or with a diffuse injury tend to do poorly on tests of abstract thinking, regardless of the mode of presentation and response. However, individuals with mild, modality-specific, or subtle dysfunction may not engage in concrete thinking generally, but do so only on those tasks that directly involve the use of an impaired modality, are highly complex, or impact on emotionally laden content.

Proverbs Test

Tests of interpretation of proverbs are among the most widely used techniques for evaluating the quality of thinking. Tests such as the Wechsler scales, the Stanford-Binet scales, and a standard Mental Status Examination include proverb interpretation items. The Proverbs Test (Gorham, 1956) formalizes the task of proverb interpretation, presenting it as an important source of information about the patient's quality of thinking. The standardization of the task reduces variations in administration and scoring biases and provides normative data that account for the difficulty level of the individual proverbs. The test has three forms, each containing 12 proverbs of essentially equal difficulty. It is administered as a written test in which the subject is asked to "tell what the proverb means rather than tell just more about it." A 3-point scoring system is used. In this system, appropriate abstract interpretations earn two points; concrete interpretation earns one point or no points if the response misses the gist of the proverb or misinterprets it. The mean scores for each form of the test do not differ significantly.

There is also a second multiple-choice version of the test that contains 40 items, each of which has four alternative explanation for the proverb. Only one of the alternatives is appropriately abstract; the remaining choices are either concrete interpretations or common misinterpretations.

TABLE 9.1   Abstract Word Test[a]

1. MISTAKE	and	LIE
2. THRIFT	and	AVARICE
3. MURDER	and	MANSLAUGHTER
4. LAZINESS	and	IDLENESS
5. COURAGE	and	BOLDNESS
6. POVERTY	and	MISERY
7. ABUNDANCE	and	EXCESS
8. TREACHERY	and	DECEIT
9. CHARACTER	and	REPUTATION
10. EVOLUTION	and	REVOLUTION

[a]Patients are asked to tell the difference between each word in the pair.

Source: Tow, P.M. (1955). *Personality changes following frontal lobe leucotomy* (p. 157). New York: Oxford University Press. Copyright © 1955, Oxford University Press. Reprinted by permission.

Scores on the Proverbs Test tend to vary with education and social class (Gorham, 1956). A study by Benton (1968) using the multiple-choice version of the test with frontal lobe–diseased patients found these patients to perform very poorly on this task, achieving a mean score of 11.4. On the multiple-choice form of the test, both schizophrenic and brain-damaged patients performed significantly more poorly than did normal control subjects; however, the two patient groups could not be differentiated from one another (Fogel, 1965).

Abstract Words Test

Tests that require abstract comparisons between two or more words can provide a sensitive measure of concrete thinking. The clinician must remember, however, that such tests are very dependent on the integrity of the patient's language skills as well as the level of verbal skills. Therefore, *patients who have even a mild dysphasia and those who have always had a low level of intellectual functioning or who have been educationally underprivileged will do more poorly on this type of test, regardless of the extent to which higher cognitive processes have been preserved.*

The Abstract Words Test (Tow, 1955) calls for comparisons between two words. The patient must tell how the words differ from one another (Table 9.1). There is no formal scoring for this test. Rather, the clinician must make a qualitative judgment as to the appropriateness of the patient's response.

A similar form of test is the Similarities subtest of the Wechsler scales.

In this test, however, the patient is required to tell how the words are the same. Scoring is done using a three-point system detailed in the WAIS-R manual. Patients tend to find this test somewhat more difficult than the Abstract Words Test noted above, as it is usually easier to tell how things differ than how they are the same.

NONVERBAL CONCEPT FORMATION

Sorting Tests

Sorting tests are by far the most common form of nonverbal tests of abstraction and concept formation. In sorting tests, the patient is asked to sort collections of objects, blocks, tokens, or other kinds of items into subgroups following instructions such as "sort out the ones that you think go together." Most sorting tests assess the patient's ability to shift concepts as well as the ability to use them effectively. The manner in which the patient proceeds usually gives an indication of his ability to form and deal with abstract concepts.

There are very few sorting tests that yield numerical scores, for *the patient's approach to the task is far more interesting than the solution for the astute clinician, who notes whether the patient sorts according to a principle, whether the principle can be formulated verbally, and whether the principle is consistently followed by the patient.*

Although sorting tests demonstrate how the patient thinks and handles certain types of abstraction problems, they have not been shown to be useful in differentiating brain-damaged from psychiatric patients (Goldstein & Scheerer, 1941). On scored tests, few significant differences have been found between the mean scores of normal controls and brain-damaged patients (Newcombe, 1969). Thus a sorting test by itself will not prove to be an effective screening test, but it can be quite useful when administered in conjunction with other tests. *When there is marked impairment of performance on a sorting test, an organically based dysfunction is likely to be present; however, marginal or questionable performance offers the clinician little useful information for differential diagnosis.*

Color Sorting Test

This simple, nonverbal sorting test by Goldstein and Scheerer (1941) consists of 61 little skeins of wool, each of which is a different combination of hue, shade, and brightness. There are about 10 skeins in each of the major colors—green, red, blue, and yellow, plus shades of gray, brown, purple, and other combined hues. The test requires the patient to (1) sort to sample; (2) match two or three different skeins, two of which are similar in hue and two in brightness; (3) explain the underlying principle of sameness in grouping of six skeins of the same hue but different shades and six skeins of different hue but the same brightness; and (4) select all of the skeins of the same hue, such as "blue" or "red," giving his reasoning for the selection. The clinician judges the patient's level and his ease of abstract thinking from both observations and the patient's accompanying explanations.

Color Form Sorting Test

Sorting tests that include a requirement to shift concepts offer more information than simple sorting tests such as the Color Sorting Test. Observation can help to clarify whether the patient's primary deficit is in sorting or in the shifting of cognitive set.

The Color Form Sorting Test (Weigl, 1941) is made up of twelve tokens or blocks colored blue, red, yellow, or green on one flat surface and all white on the opposite surface. The tokens or blocks come in three shapes (circle, square, and triangle) and are laid before the patient with the colored side up. The patient is first asked to sort the test material in any manner that is thought to be appropriate. When the patient completes the first sorting, she is then told to group them again, but in a different way. On completion of each sort, the examiner asks the patient to explain the reasoning behind the sorting that has just been completed. If the patient has difficulty in a second attempt at sorting, the examiner can offer clues, such as turning all blocks so that the white side is up if the patient's first sort was by color. If the patient performed the first sort by shape, the examiner can show the patient a single grouping formed by color and ask the patient if she can see why the blocks belong together. The inability to sort conceptually or to shift from one sorting principle to another is presumed to indicate impaired mental functioning.

A modification of this test increases the number of possible sorts to five, using thickness, size, and "suit" (a club, heart, or diamond printed at the center of the block) in addition to the four standard colors and three common shapes (DeRenzi, Faglioni, Savoiardo, & Vignolo, 1966). The first part of the test proceeds in the same manner as the original version of the test, except for a three-minute time limit. When the patient is unable to make an acceptable sort within the three-minute limit, the examiner makes each of the sorts not used by the patient and allows the patient one minute to determine the sorting principle used. Spontaneous patient sorts earn three score points each;

correct classification of the examiner's sort receives one point. Scores can range from 0 to 15. Forty control subjects were found to attain a mean score of 9.49. Patients with aphasia performed quite poorly on this modified version of the test, while patients with other types of brain injury did not appear to perform much differently from the normal group. This suggests (as do other studies of sorting tests) that left hemisphere dysfunction may result in relatively poorer performance on such tasks.

Object Sorting Test

The Object Sorting Test (Goldstein & Scheerer, 1941) is based on the same principles and generally follows the same administration procedures as are used on the block and token sorting tests, with the exception that the materials used consist of 30 common objects such as a knife, screwdriver, fork, and so forth. The objects can be grouped according to such principles as use, situation in which they can normally be found, color, pairedness, material of which the objects are made, and so on. Variations on the basic sorting task require that the patient find objects compatible with the one preselected by the examiner, to figure out a principle underlying a set of objects grouped by the examiner, to sort objects according to a category named by the examiner, or to pick out one object of an examiner selected set of objects that does not belong to the set. Most variations also require some form of verbal explanation. The Object Sorting Test allows the examiner more flexibility in the conduct of the assessment, as well as more opportunities to observe the patient's conceptual style by providing a wider range of responses than most other sorting tests. Generally, it is the qualitative aspects of the patient's responses that are considered to be important.

Vygotsky Concept Formation Test

The modified Vygotsky Concept Formation Test (Wang, 1984) is yet another sorting test. There are 22 small wooden blocks with different shapes, colors, widths, and heights. The patient is asked to sort the blocks into four groups. Feedback regarding whether the sort was correct is given following each sort. Following a completed correct sort, the patient is then asked to identify the principle by which the sort was made. As in the other tests discussed in this section, qualitative aspects of the patient's performance are important for interpretation.

Wisconsin Card Sorting Test

The Wisconsin Card Sorting Test (WCST) was devised to study "abstract behavior" and ability to "shift set" (Berg, 1948; Grant & Berg, 1948).

The patient is given a pack of 64 cards on which are printed one to four symbols—star, cross, circle, or triangle—in green, red, yellow, or blue. No two cards are identical. The patient's task is to place them, one by one, under four stimulus cards—one red triangle, two green stars, three yellow crosses, and four blue circles—according to a principle that the patient must deduce from the pattern of the examiner's responses to the patient's placement of the cards. For example, if the principle is color, the correct placement of a blue card is under four blue circles, regardless of the symbol or number, and the examiner responds accordingly. The patient just begins placing cards, and the examiner tells the patient whether the placement is correct. After a run of ten consecutive correct placements, the examiner changes the principle being used for placement, indicating the change only in the changed pattern of the "right" and "wrong" statements given to the patient. The test begins with color as the first principle, changes to form, then to number, returns to color again, and so on. The test continues until the patient has made six runs of ten correct placements, has placed more than 64 cards in one category, or uses 128 cards (Heaton, 1981).

Poor performance on this test can result from a variety of cognitive deficits. The patient may have difficulty in sorting according to category, which suggests an impaired capacity for forming abstract concepts. This difficulty most frequently occurs in patients with frontal lobe dysfunction. Perseveration (difficulty in shifting the principle used) is another common error made by patients with anterior brain damage; such performance can also be seen in patients with a long history of alcohol abuse. Parsons (1975) has also noted a third type of common error, which is referred to as "difficulty in maintaining . . . set," in which the patient may be able to form categories easily and shift set readily, but loses track of the current principle after a number of changes in the principle being used.

Of note is that Chelune and Baer (1968) present norms for children, and Spreen and Strauss (1991) offer normative data for individuals aged 60 to 94. In general, by roughly 10 years of age a child's performance is comparable with that of a young adult (Walsh, Groisser, & Pennington, 1988). Performance on the WCST appears not to significantly decline until after the age of 80 (Spreen & Strauss, 1991). A 64-item version of the WCST has been developed that has been tested on older individuals with comparable results (York Haaland, Vranes, Goodwin, & Garry, 1987).

Category Test

The Category Test (Halstead, 1947) is another test of abstraction ability. Stimulus figures, which vary in shape, size, number, intensity, color, and location and are grouped by abstract principles, are projected on a screen. The patient must figure out the principle relating stimulus subsets and respond by pressing the appropriate key on a simple keyboard. Correct responses are indicated by a bell, which sounds automatically, while incorrect responses result in a harsh buzz. The test consists of 208 items divided into seven subsets. The patient is told only that each subtest contains a single principle. Correct responses to the first few items are generally a matter of luck. However, the patient should quickly learn the pattern of bells and buzzes and modify responding by developing and testing new hypotheses until the correct principle underlying the subtest is discerned. The patient is told at the end of each subset that a new subject is about to begin in which the underlying principle may be the same or may be different from the last subset.

Subset one requires the identification of eight Roman numerals. Subtest two consists of 20 items, requiring the patient to respond to the number of items on the screen. The third section of the test contains 40 items and asks the patient to identify the position of the figure that is different from the others. Subtest 4, also 40 items, requires the patient to determine one of the four quadrants of the figure that either has a missing part or is itself missing. The fifth section contains 40 items, as does section six. Both sections use the same underlying principle, in which the salient characteristic of each stimulus is the proportion of the figure drawn with solid versus dashed lines (i.e., two quarters of the figure having solid lines requires an answer of 2; one quarter of the figure having solid lines requires a 1, etc.). The seventh and final subtest contains 20 items, many of which have been seen during the test by the patient. The patient is told that it is necessary to remember and use the principles already used to get the correct response. For the items not already used, the patient must determine the correct response in ways not totally dependent on recall of previous subtest items.

There is no time limit on the test, and although the patient is instructed to respond carefully, encouragement for prompt responding can be given. Lezak (1983) notes that the test is an excellent discriminator between brain-damaged and neurologically intact groups. A cutoff score of 50 errors is generally considered to be the point at which cognitive dysfunction is suggested. One problem with the Category Test is that the equipment required is both expensive and bulky and, thus, not very easily transportable. This has been remedied to some extent with the advent of a booklet version of the test, which appears to be as effective in its discriminative ability as the original version.

An additional problem with the Category Test is the major investment of time (and resulting frustration in the patient who is doing poorly) required when the full 208-item test is administered. Sherrill (1985, 1987) has reviewed three abbreviated versions of the Category Test; he found that a 120-item version correlated highly (0.98) with the longer version, with a small standard error of estimate. The shortened version uses all eight slides in the first subtest, the first 16 in the second subtlest, and the first 32 in each of the third, fourth, and fifth subtests. The last two subtests are omitted. This eliminates the possibility of examining memory for previous items (as is assessed by the final section of the full test); however, there is a substantial saving of time, which can be devoted to more comprehensive assessment of memory functioning.

Mattis Dementia Rating Scale

The Mattis Dementia Rating Scale (Mattis, 1976, 1988) was designed to provide a quick index of cognitive function in subjects with known or suspected dementia. It includes items similar to those employed by neurologists in bedside MSEs. The items are arranged hierarchically so that adequate performance on an initial item allows the examiner to discontinue testing within a section and assume credit can be given to the patient for adequate performance on the subsequent tasks. The subtests include measures of attention (digit span), initiation and perseveration (performing alternating movements), construction (copying designs), conceptualization (similarities), and verbal and nonverbal short-term memory (sentence recalled and design recognition).

Administration time is about 10 to 15 minutes for normal elderly individuals. Spreen and Strauss (1991) note that the test can clearly differentiate brain-impaired patients from normal elderly individuals. The instructions and scoring procedures are not as precise as would be desired; however, the test was designed as a screening device and as such works well.

ORGANIZATIONAL AND PLANNING ABILITIES

Practical and conceptual organization, ordering, and planning involve an appreciation of the categories and relationships of that which is organized, regardless of whether the organization is to be done using objects, situations, concepts, activities, or any combination of these. Cognitive flexibility to perceive alternatives is required, as well as the ability to conceptualize change from present circumstances.

There are very few formal tests of such abilities. However, the patient's handling of many standard screening tests can provide clues as to how the patient handles these conceptual functions. For instance, the layout of the Bender Visual-Motor Gestalt designs on the page indicates the patient's awareness of space usage and spatial relations. Responses to story-telling tasks can reflect the handling of sequential verbal ideas. The patient's approach to highly structured tasks, such as Block Design, provides information about whether the patient orders and plans ahead effectively, laboriously, inconsistently, or not at all.

Such information can also be obtained through the clinical interview, where questions concerning the patient's daily activities and future plans can yield indications as to organizational and planning abilities. Lezak (1975) notes that some patients, particularly those with nondominant hemisphere lesions, may give lucid and appropriate responses to questions involving organization and planning of impersonal situations or events but may show poor judgment in making unrealistic, confused, and often illogical or nonexistent plans for themselves. Additionally, such individuals may lack the judgment to recognize that they need to be able to make plans in order to remain independent.

Estimation of Premorbid Functioning

In a perfect world, all patients would be tested at some point before the onset of their brain dysfunction, preferably just prior to the event. If this were the case, then it would be a simple matter for the clinician to compare premorbid and post-morbid test data to determine the extent of dysfunction. Unfortunately, we do not live in such a world and most patients seen by clinicians do not have premorbid testing data available. Matarazzo (1990) notes that there are several clinical, medicolegal, and research situations in which knowledge of premorbid IQ is important. Several clinicians and investigators have relied on the Vocabulary and Information subtest scores of the Wechsler scales as the best indicators of premorbid functioning. Although the Vocabulary subtest is among the most resistant to change of the Wechsler subtests, performance on the test can be significantly impacted by a large range of clinical conditions (Spreen & Strauss, 1990). The Vocabulary subtest is thus likely to underestimate premorbid intelligence seriously (Crawford, 1990; Lezak,

TABLE 9.2   Barona IQ Estimate Equations

Estimated verbal IQ = 54.23 + 0.49(age) + 1.92(sex) + 4.24(race) +
   5.25(education) + 1.89(occupation) + 1.24(urban-rural residence)
Standard error of the estimate = 11.79; R = 0.62

Estimated performance IQ = 61.58 + 0.31 (age) + 1.09(sex) + 4.95(race) +
   3.75(education) + 1.54(occupation) + 0.82 (region)
Standard error of the estimate = 13.23; R = 0.49

Estimated full-scale IQ = 54.96 + 0.47(age) + 1.76(sex) + 4.71
   (race) + 5.02(education) + 1.89(occupation) + 0.59(region)
Standard error of the estimate = 12.14; R = 0.60

Variable weights (to be substituted in the preceding equations)

Sex: 1 = female; 2 = male   *Race:* 1 = other; 2 = black; 3 = white

Occupation: 1 = unskilled labor
               2 = semiskilled labor
               3 = not in labor force
               4 = skilled labor
               5 = managerial/office/clerical/sales
               6 = professional/technical

Region (U.S.): 1 = South; 2 = North Central; 3 = Western; 4 = Northeast

Residence: 1 = rural (< 2,500); 2 = urban (> 2,500)

Age: 1 = 16–17; 2 = 18–19; 3 = 20–24; 4 = 25–34; 5 = 35–44;
      6 = 45–54; 7 = 55–64 8 = 65–69; 9 = 70–74

Education (years): 1 = 0–7; 2 = 8; 3 = 9–11; 4 = 12; 5 = 13–15; 6 = 16 +

Source: Barona, A., Reynolds, C.R., & Chastain, R. (1984). A demographically based index
of pre-morbid intelligence for the WAIS-R. *Journal of Consulting and Clinical Psychology, 52,* 885–887. Adapted by permission.

1983). Although the Information subtest score can reflect a person's
general fund of knowledge, it can be misleading in patients with poor
educational background and opportunities. It has been argued that a
reading test for irregularly spelled words is a better indicator of premorbid ability as it would assess reading level achieved before the brain dysfunction (Nelson, 1982). The National Adult Reading Test (NART) was
developed in Britain to test this hypothesis. The NART is composed of
50 irregular words such as naive and debt, and has good internal and
test-retest reliability. Crawford (1990) notes that the NART does provide

a better estimate of WAIS-R IQ than Vocabulary subtest scores. NART performance does deteriorate in patients with severe cerebral dysfunction (Stebbins, Wilson, Gilley, Bernard, & Fox, 1990). Although NART performance can indeed, therefore, be affected by cognitive impairment, it may provide a lower limit to a premorbid IQ score estimate (Stebbins et al., 1990). An adaptation for use with a North American Population version of the NART was developed by Blair and Spreen (1989) and is available in the public domain for use (Spreen & Strauss, 1991).

Using demographic measures to estimate premorbid IQ functioning has also offered promising results with occupation, education, and race being the most powerful predictors (Spreen & Strauss, 1991). Numerous investigators have developed regression equations to calculate premorbid IQ (e.g., Barona, Reynolds, & Chastain, 1984; Reynolds and Gutkin, 1979). Table 9.2 shows the Baron Index formulae and variable weights. It is important to remember that the resulting indices are *estimates* of premorbid ability rather than exact indicators. An estimated premorbid Full scale IQ above 120 or less than 69 may result in significant overestimation or underestimation (Sweet, Moberg, & Tovian, 1990).

10

Neuropsychological Screening

SCREENING VERSUS SINGLE TESTS
VERSUS COMPREHENSIVE ASSESSMENTS

Comprehensive neuropsychological assessments, such as the Halstead-Reitan, the Luria-Nebraska Batteries, and the Boston Process approach have been shown for several years to be effective in differentiating brain-damaged from psychiatric and normal patients. As such, it would seem to make sense to administer a complete evaluation to every patient for whom the presence of organic dysfunction is suspected. Careful evaluation of patients seen either in private practice or in outpatient mental health clinics should identify those with brain dysfunction, allowing appropriate treatment, which otherwise might not have been considered, to be instituted. However, not all clinical psychologists or examiners have learned the necessary skills or had the training needed to competently administer and interpret a comprehensive neuropsychological assessment. These skills and knowledge can be readily acquired; however, not all clinicians are willing or able to invest the time and money necessary to develop proficiency in the art of neuropsychological diagnosis and treatment planning. Current guidelines approved by Division 40 of the American Psychological Association advise that proficiency in neuropsychology can be attained only after a minimum of one year's exclusive and full-time postdoctoral training in neuropsychology under the supervision of a qualified neuropsychologist or through a graduate degree program with a special emphasis in neuropsychology. Such training is becoming increasingly available throughout the country. There are more graduate training programs in psychology that offer a distinct emphasis in neuropsychology; however, there are still fewer than other clinical training programs. Similarly, there are few such postdoctoral training programs. The competition for the available slots at either the predoctoral or postdoctoral level is keen.

A number of highly competent clinicians feel that they can get the requisite training by attending one or another of the workshops that have proliferated in the past few years to deal with the administration and interpretation of some of the most popular neuropsychological test batteries. However, even those who offer the workshops will admit, and frequently emphasize to those in attendance, that the workshop cannot make one a competent neuropsychologist. What the clinician can gain from these workshops is a knowledge of administration techniques for a given test battery or assessment technique as well as some very basic knowledge about interpreting the results of the test. The one-, two-, or even five-day workshop does not make the clinician expert in the plethora of complex subtleties involved in brain-behavior relationships, nor is any substantial information typically given concerning the brain functions and their interrelationships that underlie manifest behaviors. Additionally, as the neuropsychology credentialing boards identify more individuals as competent practitioners, reimbursement for noncredentialed clinicians will become much more difficult to obtain.

A second reason that the private-practice clinician or the clinician working for a mental health center or private hospital may not want to perform comprehensive neuropsychological evaluations is the sheer amount of time involved. In certain circumstances a comprehensive evaluation can take up to a week, depending on the patient's physical and mental condition. More often, an evaluation will take anywhere from four to eight hours, depending on which assessment technique and supplemental tests are used. The vast majority of practicing psychologists simply do not have that amount of time to devote to a single patient. Psychologists in private practice often depend on seeing a comparatively large number of patients in any given day to earn their livelihood. For them to conduct an occasional neuropsychological evaluation that requires the devotion of a full day does not make economic sense. Practitioners working in mental health settings or in private hospitals with small staffs may be required to see far too many individuals to spend the time required for a neuropsychological evaluation of one patient.

Finally, the cost of the equipment and materials needed to conduct neuropsychological evaluations is frequently prohibitive for only occasional use. A complete Halstead-Reitan Test Battery set-up, including all equipment and materials, can cost as much as $2,500 or more at the time of this writing. The Luria-Nebraska Test Battery will cost about $425 in terms of initial costs. Both batteries now have computer-assisted scoring available, which can increase the cost still further, particularly if the clinician buys a computer. Thus, the initial investment can be great, and this cost does not include any additional test equipment or those materials that are frequently used by neuropsychologists to supplement the information from the more comprehensive batteries. By their very nature, each of the available comprehensive evaluation batteries is, in a sense, nothing more than a comprehensive screening battery that offers the possibility of generating hypotheses about the brain integrity of a patient that may in turn require further in-depth investigation with any number of other test instruments.

Thus, to perform neuropsychological evaluations, the clinician really must be willing to devote all of her professional energies to neuropsychology. It is extremely difficult to be a good "part-time" neuropsychologist without either the general clinical practice or the neuropsychological aspect of the practice suffering.

Neuropsychological screening offers a practical alternative to this, because it generally does not require much in the way of special equipment. Administration and interpretation of a screening generally requires far less time than that which is required for the more complete evaluation. Additionally, the cost in terms of both materials and personnel, as well as space, is typically a good deal less. A relatively brief, portable, and easily administered and scored battery of tests is much more practical and cost effective in those situations where the primary requirement is to differentiate those individuals who have brain-based pathology from those who do not.

Over the years a number of investigators have attempted to identify a single test that will differentiate patients with brain damage from non–brain-damaged individuals. In virtually all instances such attempts have failed and continue to do so. There is a very simple reason for this: One single test cannot possibly tap all aspects of brain functioning. There are individual tests that are exceptionally good in terms of identifying one or another form of organic dysfunction, such as the Halstead Category Test (described in Chapter 9); however, if the patient being assessed does not happen to have a dysfunction in the area being tapped by the test, but does indeed have some form of cognitive impairment, that particular patient may be inappropriately identified as non–brain-damaged. As a very simple and gross example, a patient with language disturbance will likely not be identified as impaired by the Bender Visual-Motor Gestalt; similarly, the patient with a visual-spatial processing disturbance will be classified as normal if just the Speech Perception Test is used as the screening device.

A good neuropsychological screening battery is designed to minimize the time needed for administration, scoring, and interpretation while maximizing the information gathered by briefly assessing all major cognitive functional areas. These functional areas include lateral dominance; motor functioning; auditory, tactile, and visual sensation; spatial-perceptual organization; language skills; general information; and memory processes. Furthermore, the tests included in such a battery should have as little redundancy as possible and should have been empirically demonstrated to be effective in differentiating brain-damaged from non–brain-damaged individuals. All of the tests included should be brief, easily administered, objectively scored, commonly used in clinical settings, and very portable.

What follows is a description of different screening approaches that have either been reported in professional journals or discussed at length at professional meetings. All of the batteries that will be described have been demonstrated to be effective in assisting the clinician in differential diagnosis. These screening batteries also conform, in large part, to the criteria described earlier. Most of the screenings discussed consist of tests previously described in this text. Because few of these screening techniques have a formal title, they are discussed and named after the battery developers. In the past few years, there have been several commercially available screening devices introduced. These are also discussed.

WYSOCKI AND SWEET SCREENING BATTERY

This neuropsychological screening test battery was developed by Jeffrey Wysocki and Jerry Sweet (1985). The battery consists of seven tests and requires less than one hour for administration. In the original research investigation, the average administration time for brain-damaged individuals was 55.6 minutes; for schizophrenic patients, 51.3 minutes; and for normal control subjects, 50.3 minutes.

The measures selected for the battery include: (I) the Finger Tapping Test (Halstead, 1947)—a measure of bilateral fine motor speed and dex-

TABLE 10.1   Wysocki-Sweet Screening Battery Order of Administration and Special Scoring Considerations

Test	Scoring
1. Finger Tapping	The relevant measures are the mean number of taps of the index finger of each hand.
2. Wechsler Memory Scale	Immediate and one-half hour delay scores described by Russell (1975) are used for both the Logical Memory and Visual Reproduction subtests.
3. Trail Making (Parts A and B)	The number of seconds required to complete each part.
4. Digit Symbol	The number of correctly drawn symbols in 90 seconds.
5. Stroop Color and Word Test	The age corrected raw score of the number of items correctly finished in 45 seconds on each page of the Golden (1978) version.
6. Pathognomonic Scale	Summary score for the scale obtained by adding the rating scores for each of the 34 items.
7. Spatial Relations	The Greek crosses drawn by the patient are scored using the rating scale developed by Russell, Neuringer & Goldstein (1970).

terity; (2) The Trail Making Test—Parts A and B (Armitage, 1946); (3) the Digit Symbol subtlest of the Wechsler Adult Intelligence Scale—a task assessing motor persistence, sustained attention, response speed, and visual-motor coordination; (4) the Spatial Relations component—Greek cross—of the Aphasia Screening Test (Halstead & Wepman, 1949); (5) the Pathognomonic Scale of the Luria-Nebraska Neuropsychological Battery (Golden, Hammeke, & Purisch, 1985)—a series of items from the battery that have been empirically shown to be highly sensitive to the presence of cognitive dysfunction; (6) the Stroop Color and Word Test (Stroop, 1935); and (7) the Logical Memory and Visual Reproduction subtests of the Wechsler Memory Scale (Wechsler, 1945)—here both immediate and delayed (one-half hour) recall are assessed. (It is important to note that no data have been reported using the revised version of the WMS. The original WMS should be used here.)

All tests are administered according to their normal instructions and scored in the standard manner described in the specific test manuals except where noted. The order in which the tests should be administered and specific scoring criteria are presented in Table 10.1. The order was chosen by the test developers in order to allow enough time to elapse between the immediate and delayed recall of the subtests from the Wechsler Memory Scale without presenting the competing verbal and

TABLE 10.2   Percent Correct Classification Per Test Using Cutoff Scores

Test	Brain damaged	Psychiatric patients	Normal controls
Trails A (Reitan norms)	76	72	100
(Russell norms)	88	52	84
Trails B (Reitan norms)	84	68	84
(Russell norms)	84	60	80
Tapping—Dominant (Reitan norms)	84	20	48
(Russell norms)	76	24	68
Tapping—Nondominant (Russell norms)	80	40	80
Spatial Relations (Russell norms)	67	84	96
Digit Symbol	72	72	100
Stroop (Golden Norms): Word	52	76	94
Color	72	36	96
Color-Word	48	72	96
Pathognomonic (t > 70)	40	100	100
(critical level)	75	88	100
Wechsler Memory Scale (Russell Norms)			
Semantic Short-Term	88	8	28
Semantic Delay	92	8	28
Figure Short-Term	84	40	64
Figure Delay	96	24	56

Source: Wysocki, J.J., & Sweet, J.J. (1985). Identification of brain-damaged, schizophrenic, and normal medical patients using a brief neuropsychological screening battery. *International Journal of Clinical Neuropsychology,* 7(1), 40–44. Copyright © 1985, MelNic Press. Reprinted by permission.

visual memory items found in the Pathognomonic Scale of the Luria-Nebraska Battery. The delayed recall of the Wechsler Memory Scale items is obtained one-half hour after the immediate recall portion by pausing in the administration of the Luria-Nebraska items. The remaining Pathognomonic scale items are then administered, followed by the drawing of the Greek crosses to complete the battery. On completion of the battery, the patient's performance on each measure is compared to the traditional cutoff scores for each of the tests; if a patient is impaired on six of the total of eight measures, the patient is considered to be cognitively impaired. This "6 out of 8" decision rule correctly classified 68% of the brain-damaged subjects, 84% of the schizophrenic patients as non–brain-damaged, and 100 percent of the normal control subjects of the original study sample (see Table 10.2).

The Wysocki and Sweet Screening Battery appears to be a useful screening device. It meets the criteria of brevity, ease of administration, and coverage of a broad base of neuropsychological skills and cortical functions necessary for a useful screening instrument.

Of note is the fact that this battery, as good as it may be, was only able to effect a hit rate of 68% in identification of brain-damaged individuals. This points out a problem with neuropsychological screening batteries in general—there can be a substantial number of false negatives. Often times, patients will have very subtle or highly specific deficits that a screening battery will be unable to detect. The astute clinical observer may be able to improve slightly on this figure; however, there are bound to be some impaired individuals who will not be identified. In such instances, the best strategy is to refer for comprehensive evaluation of neuropsychological functioning those patients whose screening results are suspicious but do not meet the criteria necessary to indicate cortical dysfunction.

ABBREVIATED HALSTEAD-REITAN SCREENING BATTERY, VERSION 1

Golden (1976) has offered a useful abbreviated version of the Halstead-Reitan Neuropsychological Test Battery. Version 1 of the Abbreviated Battery is somewhat more lengthy than Version 2 (described below) and requires roughly one hour for total administration. It consists of nine tests: (1) Trail Making Test, Parts A and B; (2) the Aphasia Screening Test; (3) the Seashore Rhythm Test; (4) the Speech Sounds Perception Test; (5) the Stroop Color and Word Test; and from the Wechsler Adult Intelligence Scale, the (6) Block Design; (7) Digit Symbol; (8) Similarities; and (9) Object Assembly subscales.

All of the tests in this version of the Abbreviated Battery are administered in the generally accepted manner. Scoring for the Wechsler scale subtests requires use of the age-corrected scale scores. For the Trail Making Test, the total combined time to complete Part A and Part B. in seconds, is the score to be used. On the Stroop Color and Word Test, three scores are generated—number of items completed on the word, color, and combined word-color pages. Scores on both the Speech Sounds Perception Test and Seashore Rhythm Test are the number of incorrect response on each test. The Aphasia Screening Test is scored in accordance with the technique of Russell, Neuringer, and Goldstein (1970), which assigns different weights to each item based on its importance.

All test scores are then compared against what are considered to be cutting scores for performance within the normal range (see Table 10.3).

TABLE 10.3   Cutting Scores for the Tests in the Golden (1976) Abbreviated Version of the Halstead-Reitan Battery

Test	Cutting Score[a]
Aphasia Screening Test	> 6 points
Speech Sounds Perception Test	> 7 errors
Seashore Rhythm Test	> 5 errors
Trail Making Test—Part A	> 33 seconds
Trial Making Test—Part B	> 87 seconds
Stroop—Word Page	< 87 items
—Color Page	< 59 items
—Color-Word Page	< 32 items
WAIS—Block Design	< 9 scale score
—Similarities	< 9 scale score
—Digit Symbol	< 9 scale score
—Object Assembly	< 9 scale score

[a]Indicating impaired performance.

Source: Golden, C.J. (1976). The identification of brain damage by an abbreviated form of the Halstead-Reitan Neuropsychological Battery. *Journal of Clinical Psychology, 32,* 821–826. Copyright © 1976, Clinical Psychology Publishing Company. Adapted by permission.

An impairment index is obtained by calculating the percentage of tests that fall within the normal or impaired range. If the performance falls within the normal range for a specific test, a value of 0 is assigned. If the patient's performance is within the impaired range on a specific test, a value of 1 is assigned. It is then a simple matter to determine if a majority of the test scores have values in the impaired range. If this is the case, there is a reasonable probability that the patient has organic dysfunction.

Golden (1976) also developed a somewhat more accurate (and complex) method of determining whether a patient's test performance on the Abbreviated Battery, Version 1, falls within the impaired or normal range. A single score for each patient's performance is obtained by multiplying the patient's score on each measure by the appropriate, empirically derived coefficient listed in Table 10.4.

All derived products are then summed. If the patient's derived score is greater than 210, impairment is indicated. This technique yielded a hit rate of 71.9% with an amazingly high correct identification rate of 97% of individuals with left hemisphere damage in the original research conducted with the Abbreviated Battery, Version 1. Alternatively, the patient's individual test score index (0 or 1) can be multiplied by the general test index listed in Table 10.4, and the resulting products can be summed and compared with the cutoff score of 210.

TABLE 10.4 Golden Abbreviated Battery Unstandardized Coefficients for Differentiation of Brain Damaged and Normal Performance

Test	Coefficient	Index
Seashore Rhythm Test	3.1	41.7
Speech Sounds Perception Test	1.2	5.8
Trail Making Test—Part A	0.3	−26.8
Trail Making Test—Part B	−0.2	138.7
Aphasia Screening Test	2.0	−18.8
WAIS—Similarities	1.1	−29.2
—Digit Symbol	−0.5	66.0
—Object Assembly	17.2	48.4
—BlockDesign	−4.4	126.1
Stroop—Word	−0.5	−35.1
—Color	−1.2	−13.6
—Color-Word	−0.1	−19.7

Source: Golden, C.J. (1976). The identification of brain damage by an abbreviated form of the Halstead-Reitan Neuropsychological Battery. *Journal of Clinical Psychology, 32,* 821–826. Copyright © 1976, Clinical Psychology Publishing Company. Adapted by permission.

ABBREVIATED HALSTEAD-REITAN SCREENING BATTERY, VERSION 2

In 1978, an abbreviated version of the Halstead-Reitan Neuropsychological Test Battery was reported in the literature (Erickson, Calsyn, & Scheupbach, 1978). Based on that original investigation, McNamara, Wechsler, and Munger (1984) studied the utility of the Abbreviated Battery. The Abbreviated Battery is quite short and is easily administered in well under one hour.

The screening device consists of four basic tests: (1) the Trail Making Test (Parts A and B scored in accord with Russell et al., 1970; (2) the Aphasia Screening Test (Russell, 1975, scoring); and the Wechsler Adult Intelligence Scale (3) Block Design and (4) Digit Symbol subtest scale scores. Standard administration and scoring methods are applied to each of the tests. The patient's performance is then compared to the following cutoff scores. An average impairment rating is calculated as follows:

Step 1:
Total Impairment Score = 27.338

+ (1.043 × Trail Making A plus B Russell*
  rating)
+ (-0.655 × Block Design Scale Score)
+ (1.695 × Russell Aphasia Error Rating)
+ (-0.959 x Digit Symbol Scale Score)

(Refers to Russell, Neuringer, and Goldstein, 1970.)

Step 2
Average Impairment Rating = Total Impairment Score / 12

If the average impairment rating is equal to or greater then 1.55, than impairment is suggested. Using this technique, McNamara and associates (1984) were able to classify correctly 84 % of the original 90 cases studied into impaired and nonimpaired groups. Their work also found a high degree of association between the standard Reitan impairment index calculated from performance on the complete Halstead-Reitan Battery and the average impairment index obtained from the Abbreviated Battery.

The results obtained in the investigation of McNamara and associates (1984) indicate that the Abbreviated Battery may be a useful screening technique that requires comparatively little in terms of cost as well as administration time. As is the case with all the neuropsychological screening batteries mentioned in this chapter, additional research is needed; however, the potential clinical utility of this Abbreviated Battery is quite promising.

WECHSLER ADULT INTELLIGENCE SCALE AS A NEUROPSYCHOLOGICAL SCREENING INSTRUMENT

A Historical Perspective

The majority of early studies of the neuropsychological diagnostic possibilities of the Wechsler scales were conducted with mixed organic populations with no regard for the nature, extent, or location of lesions. A consistent pattern of subtest scores was noted from these studies, in which subtests requiring immediate memory, concentration, response speed, and abstract concept formation were most likely to show the effects of brain damage. The performances of these same patients on tests of previously learned information and verbal associations were found to be the least affected. While recognizing the inconsistency of relationships between Wechsler subtest score patterns and various kinds of lesions, Wechsler and others noted the similarities between these subtests, which are apparently sensitive to brain damage, and the subtests most prone to age-related changes. Efforts to apply this seeming relationship to questions of differential diagnosis resulted in a variety of formulae and ratios that were used to classify patients into global diagnostic categories. To date, none of these formulas or ratios have demonstrated any consistently valid efficacy.

Wechsler (1945) developed a deterioration quotient (DQ), which was designed to allow the examiner to compare scores on tests that tended not to be affected with aging ("Hold" tests) with those scores thought to decline with advancing age ("Don't Hold" tests). The assumption that Wechsler made was that cognitive deterioration indices that exceeded the normal limits implied early cortical deterioration, an abnormal organically-based process, or both. For the WAIS the DQ was calculated using age-corrected scores in a comparison of the "Hold" tests (Information, Vocabulary, Object Assembly, and Picture Completion) with the "Don't Hold" tests (Digit Span, Digit Symbol, Similarities, and Block Design), using the following formula:

$$DQ = (\text{Hold-Don't Hold}) / \text{Hold}$$

If the resulting deterioration quotient exceeded 0.10, possible dysfunction was suspected; while if the DQ exceeded 0.20, definite impairment was indicated. Unfortunately, *there is a large body of research indicating that this system simply does not work* and results in 25% to 57% incorrect classification of patients. Over the years, several investigators have attempted to develop similar formula systems using data from the WAIS, with varying degrees of success. However, *no one system has ever held up under cross-validation or been consistently accurate in identifying organically impaired individuals to the exclusion of other patient and normal populations.*

Pattern Analysis of the WAIS and Cognitive Dysfunction

The subtests of the WAIS are differentially affected by different types and locations of brain dysfunction (Golden, 1979). Recognition of this fact has generated a good deal of research to find patterns of subtest scores that signify different brain lesions. This pattern can then be matched against patterns expected in different kinds of brain injury. If the pattern matches what would be expected in a given brain injury, then the patient is likely to suffer from localized dysfunction in that portion of the brain.

The most ambitious use of the WAIS for this purpose was reported by McFie (1975). In this report, McFie outlines the basic patterns that can be expected in different types of localized brain injuries. Left frontal lesions tend to be characterized by a decrease on Digit Span with an attendant mild loss, or no loss, in the verbal IQ score. Such injuries will also be accompanied by a deficit in verbal associative learning. Right frontal dysfunction appears to lead to performance decrements in Picture Arrangement, memory tasks involving designs, and occasionally in Digits Backward. Left temporal injury frequently produces losses on Similarities and Digit Span, while damage to right temporal areas of the brain can result in a drop on Picture Arrangement as well as Memory for Designs. Meier and French (1966) have also suggested that a decline on Object Assembly can be seen with right temporal lesions. Lesions of the left varietal lobes will generally cause poor performance on Arithmetic, Digit Span, Block Design, and sometimes Similarities (Mahan, 1976). Right varietal dysfunction will often affect performance on Memory for Designs, Block Design, and Picture Arrangement.

Diffuse injuries typically will lead to declines on most of the suggests that have been found to be sensitive to brain injury—Digit Span, Arithmetic, Picture Arrangement, Object Assembly, Block Design, and Digit Symbol. It should be noted that Digit Symbol can be affected by a variety of factors and is frequently depressed even in normal individuals. If the subcortical areas have been damaged, those subtests affected tend to be the ones with a strong motor component, such as Digit Symbol, Block Design, Object Assembly, and Picture Arrangement, in that order (Golden, 1979).

Dysfunction resulting from injury to the brain early in childhood, particularly if the injury occurs prior to the age of two years, will show a considerably different pattern of scores from that seen with adult injuries. As a rule, the patient will have a full-scale IQ below 80. Those tests that traditionally have been considered as "Hold" tests (Information, Vocabulary, Comprehension) will typically be among the lowest scores on the WAIS. This pattern results from the inability of the child with early brain damage to take full advantage of educational opportunities and from the day-to-day learning that occurs in childhood. Frequently the scores that are highest in these patients will be on Digit Span, Picture Completion, Arithmetic, and Block Design. Recognition of such a pattern can allow the clinician to differentiate between comparatively early brain injury and damage that has occurred later in the patient's life.

It must be emphasized that, as a test of organicity, the WAIS-R is really not sensitive enough to be used alone. If the WAIS-R is combined with a test of visual memory, such as the Benton Visual Retention Test, it can be somewhat useful as a screening instrument; however, in a good many cases, the WAIS-R is not diagnostically accurate enough to be used in the differentiation of brain-damaged versus non–brain-damaged groups.

THE WAIS-R AS A NEUROPSYCHOLOGICAL INSTRUMENT

Most recently, there has been a new addition to the literature concerning the WAIS-R. The WAIS-R as a Neuropsychological Instrument (WAIS-R-NI) (Kaplan, Fein, Morris, & Delis, 1991) has been introduced as a supplement to the WAIS-R to provide information that is useful as part of a comprehensive psychological evaluation, neuropsychological evaluation, or an initial screening to determine the need for a more comprehensive evaluation. The WAIS-R-NI contains new subtests and modifications for WAIS-R subtest administration, recording, and scoring. (If the clinician already owns the WAIS-R, the WAIS-R-NI kit can be purchased separately. The WAIS-R is required to use the WAIS-R-NI segments.) Most of the changes still allow for obtaining standard scores. The more in-depth procedure allows for a finer analysis of a patient's behavior and cognitive functioning. A cognitive function profile can be generated from the test results that allow for a graphic representation of an individual's performance pattern. The changes in the WAIS-R include a multiple choice answer format that can be used following the standard administration of the Information, Vocabulary, Comprehension, and Similarities subtests. The Arithmetic subtest also has been modified to offer an alternative method of administration that can help in differentiating among problems in memory, reasoning, computation or visual-spatial deficits, all of which can contribute to poor performance on this subtest. A Symbol Copy task has been added to allow for a better measure of copying speed as well as allow for a clearer picture of problems in visual-spatial processing as assessed by the Digit Symbol subtest. Other new subtests include a Sentence Arrangement task, which allows for assessing a patient's ability to sequence meaningful verbally-based information and a Spatial Span task, which assesses aspects of visual memory processing. Detailed administration and scoring procedures are presented in the manual as is much information for interpretation.

The WAIS-R-NI represents the first major modification designed to use the Wechsler Intelligence Scales as a tool for directly investigating brain function. As such, it is a significant step forward. As an in-depth evaluation instrument, the WAIS-R-NI can be extremely useful; however, a complete administration can be very lengthy. Comparatively little data are available as of this writing discussing the use of the instrument in the described manner for a screening. Limited clinical use as a screening device by one of the authors suggests that there is much potential in the WAIS-R-NI. Additional empirical and clinical research is being conducted to investigate this approach fully.

The results of a recent meta-analysis of the relative sensitivity of neuropsychological screening tests indicated that a brief, highly sensitive and functionally wide-ranging neuropsychological test battery can be assembled (Chouinard & Braun, 1993). In this study, the authors metaanalyzed the literature to assemble empirical evidence of the existence of statistically significant sensitive screening tests across an equivalently wide range of functional domains in response to the recommended NIMH neuropsychological test battery (Butters et al., 1990; Adams & Heaton, 1990), which requires 7 to 9 hours for administration. The tests recommended in the NIMH battery are presented in Table 10.5. Chouinard and Braun (1993) offer a grouping of these screening tests by functioning as presented below in Table 10.6. Several common and frequently used tests were not included in the study as research reports concerning the utility of the tests was insufficiently frequent for inclusion in the study. The authors also strongly caution that the study results do not offer a proposal for a test battery that should be applied in all cases. This is largely because many of these tests have unusual psychometric properties that may call into question the reliability and validity of the tests in certain instances. Again, we must caution the reader against blindly creating a battery out of these specific, or other, tests without first fully investigating their clinical utility and statistical properties.

AUTOMATED NEUROPSYCHOLOGICAL ASSESSMENT METRICS

The Automated Neuropsychological Assessment Metrics (ANAM) tests developed by Reeves and colleagues (D. Reeves, personal communication, August 1993) builds on earlier neuropsychological assessment studies conducted at Walter Reed Army Medical Center, the National Naval Medical Center in Bethesda, The National Aeronautics and Space Administration, and the North Atlantic Treaty Organization. All tests are administered via computer and have been demonstrated to be applicable for general clinical and bedside testing as well as while patients are un-

TABLE 10.5   Cognitive Categories and Tests of the NIMH Battery

B.   Attention
    1. Digit Span (WMS-R)
    2. Visual Span (WMS-R)
C.   Speed of Processing
    1. Sternberg Search Task
    2. Simple and Choice Reaction Times
    3. Paced Auditory Serial Addition Test (PASAT)
D.   Memory
    1. California Verbal Learning Test (CVLT)
    2. Working Memory Test
    3. Modified Visual Reproduction Test (WMS)
E.   Abstraction
    1. Category Test
    2. Trail Making Test, Parts A and B
F.   Language
    1. Boston Naming Test
    2. Letter and Category Fluency Test
G.   Visual-spatial
    1. Embedded Figures Test
    2. Money's Standardized Road Map Test of Direction Sense
    3. Digit Symbol Substitution
H.   Construction Abilities
    1. Block Design Test
    2. Tactual Performance Test
I.   Motor Abilities
    1. Grooved Pegboard
    2. Finger Tapping Test
    3. Grip Strength

dergoing neurosurgery. The tests are designed to be culture fair, and all are in the public domain, thus avoiding potential copyright infringement problems.

The ANAM battery consists of measures of fatigue, simple reaction time, choice reaction time, procedural reaction time, spatial processing (both simultaneous and successive), and tracking. Additionally, a variety of measures of memory are included (e.g., the Sternberg Memory Search Task), and a mood a scale is available. As noted earlier, the tests are computer administered and require little training for the clinician. The instructions are fairly self-explanatory. The response keys the patient is initially required to use to respond to test items do not make intuitive sense; however, these are very easily changed. The software has excellent documentation available. (The ANAM software is available from the Office of Military Performance Assessment Technology (OMPAT), Divi-

TABLE 10.6   Categories and Tests Identified by the Meta-Analysis

1. Speed of Processing
   a. Choice Reaction Time
   b. Simple Reaction Time
2. Attention and Concentration
   a. Stroop Color and Word Test
   b. Digit Span
3. Motor Abilities
   a. Grooved Pegboard
   b. Finger Tapping
   c. Grip Strength
4. Complex Visual Perception
   a. Facial Recognition
   b. Line Orientation
5. Memory
   a. WMS-R Visual Delayed Memory
   b. WMS-R Verbal Delayed Memory
   c. Duration of Delay
6. Constructional Abilities
   a. Rey Complex Figure
   b. Block Design
7. Language
   a. Verbal Fluency (semantic)
   b. Boston Naming Test
8. Problem Solving
   a. Tactual Performance Test
   b. Trail Making Test, Parts A and B
   c. Category Test
9. Executive Functions
   a. Design Fluency
   b. Wisconsin Card Sorting Test
   c. Verbal Fluency (phonologic)

Source: Chouinard, M.J., & Braun, C.M.J. (1993). A meta-analysis of the relative sensitivity of neuropsychological screening tests. *Journal of Clinical and Experimental Neuropsychology, 15,* 591–607.

sion of Neuropsychiatry, Walter Reed Army Medical Institute of Research, Washington, DC 20307-5100. The software also can be downloaded via the OMPAT bulletin board, which is available 24 hours a day by dialing 301-427-5396 [< 9,600 Baud] or 301-427-5279 [> 9,600 Baud]. The needed communication parameters are 8-bit word, 1-stop bit, no parity, full duplex.)

Reeves (1993) considers the ANAM tests to be particularly useful in situations in which repeated measures testing is required (for example, serial testing to monitor recovery after a traumatic brain injury, or presurgical and postsurgical intervention). Summary graphs of tests results can be used to explain changes in performance across time to patients and family members.

At the current time, there is comparatively little normative data available for the ANAM. The tests, therefore, must be used and interpreted with great care. The test developers suggest that the data are best used for ideographic assessment. A national data base is being compiled at the Missouri Institute of Mental Health and it is expected that normative data tables will be available in the future. The ANAM battery blends traditional neuropsychological assessment with the approaches of experimental cognitive psychology. As such, it holds great promise as the next generation of neuropsychological measures.

BARRY REHABILITATION INPATIENT SCREENING OF COGNITION

The Barry Rehabilitation Inpatient Screening of Cognition (BRISC) (Barry et al., 1989; Barry, 1991) was developed because of a perceived clinical need to provide reliable information to physicians and rehabilitation treatment teams after a brief consultation with brain-injured patients. Many items were derived from existing instruments with the intent to consolidate those that have been found to be most useful in treatment planning. The BRISC is divided into eight functional categories providing the clinician with a broad sample of cognitive functions in approximately 30 minutes. The BRISC can be used as a more general screening device as well as failure on a significant number of items can reflect the presence of significant brain impairment, which may require further investigation.

The first category, Reading, was designed to separate commonly found problems with visual acuity from visual language processing. A variety of visual-motor, oral-motor reading, and comprehension problems may be inferred from the patient's performance on the five items comprising this section.

The second category, Design Copy, requires the patient to copy five common geometrical shapes. These shapes also become the basis for immediate and delayed spatial memory sections when assessing memory. In the Verbal Concepts portion of the BRISC, word pairs are presented and the patient is asked how each pair is alike and how the words in the pair differ. Additionally, these words are used in the memory section to assess immediate and delayed verbal memory. The fourth category, Orientation, requires the patient to provide typical orientation information. Category V, Mental Imagery, was included as individuals with brain dysfunction often have difficulty in accurately reporting internal visual representations. In this section, the patent is asked to recite the entire alphabet and then only those letters with curves in them when printed in capital letters. The sixth category, Mental Control, includes a standard digit-span task (including both forward and backward recitation), as well as a sequential alternation task that is comparable with an oral version of Trail Making, Part B. A measure of Verbal Fluency comprises section 7. The patient is asked to generate lists of groceries and clothing. The final section, Memory, includes four measures of incidental memory for the previously seen geometrical designs and word pairs that were presented earlier.

The initial investigation demonstrated good concurrent validity with accepted measures of cognitive functioning as well as acceptable reliability. A total score of 135 is possible on the BRISC. Scores below 120 points are considered to be indicative of impaired functioning. It is important for the clinician to remember that the BRISC originally was designed for use with and standardized on an inpatient population. Normative data were gathered from normal adults. While the concepts which underlie the items can be reasonably expected to apply for non-hospitalized individuals, to date no data concerning the validity of the BRISC as a screening measure are available, and, thus, the BRISC should be used judiciously.

NEUROBEHAVIORAL COGNITIVE STATUS EXAMINATION

The Neurobehavioral Cognitive Status Examination (NCSE) (Kiernan, Mueller, Langston, & van Dyke, 1987; Mueller, Kiernan, & Langston, 1988; Schwamm, van Dyke, Kiernan, Merrin, & Mueller, 1987; Yazdanfar, 1990) was developed in the mid-1980s as a response to a growing need for a brief assessment of different areas of cognitive functioning. The authors reject the use of a MSE and other comparable measures that quantify cognitive status with a single score in favor of a multivariate approach that provides indices for different functional abilities. Instead of evaluating "organicity" per se, the NCSE was therefore designed to assess neuropsychological functions in a brief manner. The NCSE addresses five major domains of cognitive functioning—language (comprehension, repetition, and naming), construction, memory, calculation, and reasoning (similarities and judgment)—as well as overall level of consciousness, orientation, and attention. It incorporates a screen as well as a metric approach and allows for the development of a profile of the patient's cognitive functioning in different areas. On the sections with a screening item, if it is passed, the clinician can move to the next section without administering the items that compose the metric portion. Total administration time rarely exceeds 20 to 30 minutes. The test manual provides some reliability and validity data, as well as some limited normative data.

Section I of the NCSE is a simple assessment of level of consciousness. If the patient is not fully alert, the test should be discontinued as interpretation is not meaningful. Section II consists of traditional Orientation questions which the patient must answer. In section III, Attention, the patient is asked to perform a digit span (forward) task. The second portion of this section requires the patient to repeat four words just related to him or her. For the four-part Language section of the NCSE, section IV, a speech sample is obtained in part one from the patient by asking her to describe the action in a picture. Although no score is given for this, it allows for a qualitative assessment of the patient's spontaneous speech. Comprehension (part 2) is next assessed in this section. The patient is asked to perform one-, two-, and three-step tasks in response to verbal commands. Oral language comprehension and complex motor praxis are both involved in this test. For part 3, the clinician asks the patient to repeat phrases and sentences after oral presentation. Finally, in part 4, Naming, the patient is asked to name objects and pictures of objects to visual confrontation. Section V of the NCSE assesses Construction ability. The screen task involves concentration, visual memory, and construction ability. The patient is presented with a complex visual figure to be drawn after a 10 second presentation. In the metric section, the patient is asked to perform a block design task. Section VI investigates memory. The patient is asked to recall the four words presented in an earlier portion of the NCSE. If needed, the patient is presented with category prompts and, finally, verbally presented recognition lists. The Calculations section (VII) consists of a series of arithmetic computations to be performed mentally after oral presentation. Section VII, Reasoning, is divided into two parts. Part A, Similarities, is basically the same as the task of the same name on the Wechsler scales. The patient is presented with two words and required to tell how they are alike. Part B, Judgment, consists of practical judgment questions in the form, "What would you do if . . . ?" All responses are scored according to generally clear criteria presented in the manual. Section scores are summed and then plotted on the front of the test booklet. Preliminary research conducted with the NCSE suggests that it is a highly useful screening device and worthy of further clinical investigation (e.g., Costello, Bieliauskas, & Terpenning, 1992; Fields, Starratt, Fishman, Cisewski, & Coffey, 1993).

COGNITIVE COMPETENCY TEST

The Cognitive Competency Test (CCT) (Wang, 1990; Wang & Ennis, 1986; Wang, Ennis, & Copeland, 1987) was developed to assess directly an individual's cognitive competency in maintaining safe and independent living. Although not a neuropsychological screening device per se, it is believed that the CCT can be a valuable instrument in a clinician's armamentarium. The CCT incorporates the concept of multidimensionality of cognitive skill and uses a practical approach by simulating daily living skills. The broad range of skills tapped by the CCT offers the clinician a more representative picture of the cognitive competency of the patient.

The CCT consists of eight subtests, each of which measures a different behavioral-cognitive domain. Subtest 1, Personal Information, asks the patient to write information on a printed form resembling application forms used by banks and public agencies. If the patient is unable to write as a function of a specific motor problem or an agraphia, the information can be obtained verbally by the examiner. Card Arrangement, Subtest 2, uses five sets of cards to demonstrate the sequences of baking a pie, preparing a meal, sweeping the floor, and doing laundry. The patient is required to arrange the cards into the proper order to demonstrate his or her knowledge of the sequence of actions needed to perform daily activities. Picture Interpretation, Subtest 3, is designed to require the patient to make use of visually presented information to come to conclusions about interactions of the individuals in the picture. The design of the task is such that the patient must logically deduce events either preceding or following the situation presented in the picture. Memory, Subtest 4, has two sections, immediate and delayed recall. The items to be remembered are practical with a day to day relevance: a grocery list, current prices for bus fare and stamps, and an appointment. Administration simulates real-life situations by providing the opportunity for rehearsal through repeated presentation and delayed recall with interference. Practical Reading Skills, Subtest 5, consists of 10 pictures depicting different settings such as a railway station, supermarket entrance, telephone directory, and so on. The patient is required to read various simple labels and signs in order to answer a question about the picture. Management of Finances, Subtest 6, is designed to determine the ability to handle the specifics and the mechanics of financial

TABLE 10.7 CCT Score Classification

Average Total Score (%)	Level of cognitive competency and functional independence
80 and higher	Total independence
70–79	Mostly independent; occasional assistance may be required
56–69	Partial independence; partial and structured assistance is required
45–55	Varying from partial and structured assistance to stand-by supervision
31–44	Mostly dependent; stand-by supervision required
30 and lower	Total dependence

Source: Wang, P.L. (1990). Assessment of cognitive competency. In. D.E. Tupper & K.D. Cicerone (Eds.), *The neuropsychology of everyday life: Assessment and basic competencies*. Boston: Kluwer Academic Publishers. Adapted by permission.

matters and requires a good deal of accuracy on the part of the patient in executing the details of the test. The task includes sorting mail, deciding bills to be paid, writing a check, and computing a balance. Verbal Reasoning and Judgment, Subtest 7, consists of 10 questions intended to assess the patient's understanding of strategies needed for self-preservation and safety judgment. Route Learning and Spatial Orientation, Subtest 8, consists of maps with different landmarks, assesses specific types of memory (locations and names of landmarks as well as memory for routes), and directional orientation and spatial judgment. The task requires the use of visual-spatial memory and verbal memory to a lesser extent for successful completion.

The scores of the eight subtests are summed to yield an average total score (percentage form) that the authors report to be a robust indicator of the level of cognitive competency. Cut-off scores also are provided for each subtest to assist in the identification of strengths and weaknesses in various cognitive skills. The range of scores and identified competency level is presented in Table 10.7. The initial validation data look good. Comprehensive research is underway to evaluate both the legal and psychological efficacy of the CCT.

MINI-INVENTORY OF RIGHT BRAIN INJURY

The Mini-Inventory of Right Brain Injury (MIRBI) (Pimental & Kingsbury, 1989) is a 27 item instrument that was designed to be used as a tool for screening cognitive deficits associated with right-hemisphere lesions. As originally conceived, the MIRBI is a relatively rapid screening that highlights areas of deficient processing and allows clinicians to identify neurocognitive domains in need of further examination using a more comprehensive battery. Test results also can assist in delineating for referral sources of a treatment team potential areas needing immediate treatment emphasis. The items of the MIRBI assess a variety of right-hemisphere processes as detailed in Table 10.8.

The MIRBI was originally normed on a patient population with well-documented right- or left-hemisphere cerebral vascular accidents, as well as normal individuals. The test has good initial and cross-validation data (Knight, Pimental, Miller, & McWilliams, 1990; Pimental & Knight, 1991). The MIRBI total score discriminated normal controls from documented lesion groups with a hit rate of 99.97% in the original validation study and an average hit rate of about 90% in the cross-validation. The MIRBI's short time for administration, portability, and item content selected for sensitivity to right brain injury combine for an initial screening device of high utility.

ASSESSMENT OF COGNITIVE SKILLS

The Assessment of Cognitive Skills (ACS) (Powell et al., 1991) is designed as a self-administered, computerized neuropsychological screening device that has been developed to detect age-inappropriate cognitive changes. The ACS was originally developed in such a manner as to emphasize the process-oriented approach to neuropsychological assessment. The decision to computerize the ACS was based on seven considerations: ease of administration and standardization; cost effectiveness; capacity for multiple simultaneous administrations; the precise quantification of reaction time and problems-solving strategies; the ability to present an easier or more difficult item based on the success or failure on the preceding item; the capacity to terminate the presentation of a subtest when a patient has reached the limits of her abilities; and ease of governing alternative forms. The test consists of 21 subtests that cover five general cognitive domains: reactivity and attention; verbal and visual memory; visual-spatial perception; mental calculation; and conceptualization and abstract reasoning (see Table 10.9).

The ACS yields three scores: the total score (maximum = 207), subtest scores, and response times. In addition to a patient's response choice, reaction times to that choice also are obtained. Additionally, on those subtests that have a multiple-choice response format, quantitative and

TABLE 10.8 MIRBI General Item Content

Visual scanning
Finger naming
Stereognosis
Two-point discrimination
Unilateral neglect

Reading comprehension
General reading skills
Spontaneous writing
Dictated writing
Cursive *M*s & *W*s
Serial 7s
11:10 Clock Drawing

Expressing happy voice
Expressing sad voice

Understanding humor
Conversation comprehension
Verbal absurdities
Proverb 1
Proverb 2

qualitative data can be derived. The response alternatives were developed in an attempt to identify error patterns that may be associated with different brain-impaired populations. In the original standardization study, 1,104 volunteer physicians ranging in age from 28 to 92 years were studied, and it was noted that ACS scores decreased monotonically with increasing age. The initial reliability studies indicated adequate stability and consistency, as well as reasonable test-retest reliability. The initial research also investigated the impact of emotion states on ACS performance. It was found that the ACS scores were not significantly impacted by the emotional states of depression, anxiety, and anger. The original predictive validation studies reported by Powell et al. (1991) indicated a predictive accuracy of about 90% overall, which is a good deal higher than that of numerous other established neuropsychological instruments. A cross-validation study (Cimino, Behner, Cattarin, & Tantleff, 1991) resulted in an agreement in predicting impairment using both the ACS and a comprehensive neuropsychological test battery of 75%. Thus, the research conducted with the ACS to date suggests that the ACS is a psychometrically sound and valid device for screening of

TABLE 10.9   ACS Subtests

I.   Tests of Reactivity and Attention
   A. Reactivity
         Reaction Times 1
         Reaction Times 2
   B. Attention Span, Vigilance, Response Inhibition, Perseverance
         Numbers Forward
         Numbers Reversed
         Alikes
         Alphabet
II. Tests of Memory
   A. Verbal Memory
         Address
         Story 1 (immediate recall)
         Story 1 (delayed recall)
         Story 2 (immediate recall)
         Story 2 (delayed recall)
         Wordlist 1
         Wordlist 2
   B. Visual Memory
         Tic Tac 1
         Tic Tac 2
III. Tests of Visuospatial Perception
         Cubes
         Clocks 1
         Clocks 2
IV. Tests of Mental Calculation
         Math
V.   Tests of Abstract Reasoning and Conceptualization
         Analogies
         Object Match

neuropsychological function. Additional cross-validation and clinical studies will likely further demonstrate the utility of this device.

MICROCOG: ASSESSMENT OF COGNITIVE FUNCTIONING

MicroCog (M. Ledbetter, The Psychological Corporation, personal communication, September 1993) is the commercially available, extended version of the ACS. The instrument is intended as a screening device and a diagnostic tool for use either independently or as part of a comprehensive assessment. Two forms of the test are available. The Standard Form consists of 18 subtests and can be completed in roughly 1 hour, whereas the Short Form comprises 12 subtests with an administration time of about 30 minutes. As was the case with the ACS, MicroCog is computer administered and scored. Normative scores that are derived from a nationally representative sample of adults are available for each subtest. The device was specifically designed to be sensitive to detecting cognitive impairment across a wide age range and considers levels of premorbid intellectual functioning by providing age- and education-adjusted norms.

MicroCog is divided into five cognitive domains with a number of subtests in each domain. Domain 1 involves attention and mental control and specifically assesses immediate attention span, vigilance, concentration, perseverance, and resistance to interference. Domain 2 assesses memory—short-term, delayed verbal memory, as well as recall and recognition. Domain 3 involves the assessment of reasoning and calculations and consists of two reasoning subtests—verbal and visual—as well as a match calculations section that taps the ability to perform mental computations. Domain 4 includes the examination of visual-spatial processing including visual recognition, visual memory for spatial arrays, and visuoperceptual analysis of clock faces. The final domain assesses simple reaction time.

MicroCog uses a process-oriented approach to assessment as well as an underlying theoretical orientation emphasizing a distinction among major neurocognitive domains and their underlying distributed cortical networks. This allows for an assessment of cognitive functions, such as attention, memory, language, visual-spatial processes, abstraction, and cognitive flexibility. The demonstration version of the program available at the time this is being written (presented at the annual meeting of the American Psychological Association, August 1993) was impressive in its depth and breadth of coverage for a screening device. It is easy to operate and can be administered with comparatively little training. It is important to remember, however, that as is the case with all psychological tests, the clinician using this device should be appropriately qualified. The output generated by the test provides summary scores as well as comparison with reference groups. The test developers also note that MicroCog specifically can be used clinically for diagnosis and identification of neurocognitive impairment; early identification of dementias and degenerative conditions; identification and screening of individuals at risk for cognitive impairment; quantification of severity of cognitive impairment; differential diagnosis (e.g., cortical vs. subcortical involvement, depression vs. pseudodementia vs. dementia); age-related vs. non–age-related cognitive decline; assessment of the efficacy of certain interventions; qualitatively describe aspects of cognitive functioning; and objectively monitor disease course.

To use the program, the clinician must have an appropriate IBM-type personal computer, purchase the platform software from which the program must be run, purchase the program software, and then license the software on a per administration basis. Thus, MicroCog could potentially involve a substantial initial investment as well as continuing costs for additional administrations of the device.

Overall, the program is impressive and will likely be a highly useful device for screening for brain impairment; however, it will be a while before independent cross-validations are completed. The clinician should be careful in the use of this device until additional work is completed.

THE MIDDLESEX ELDERLY ASSESSMENT OF MENTAL STATE

The Middlesex Elderly Assessment of Mental State (MEAMS) (Golding, 1989) has been designed as one of a proliferation of devices to assess cognitive functioning in the elderly. As is the case with the Dementia Rating Scale (Mattis, 1988) discussed earlier, the MEAMS was designed to offer the clinician a quick screening of cognitive functioning in older individuals to determine if additional assessment is required. Specifically, the MEAMS assesses gross impairment of specific cognitive skills in the elderly to differentiate between functional illness and organically-based cognitive impairments. The test consists of 12 tasks and taps a wide range of cognitive domains including orientation, language, calculation, construction, visual processing, memory and limited motor functioning. A listing of the specific content areas is presented in Table 10.10. There are two alternate forms that can be used, allowing the clinician to do test-retest to determine gross changes over time. Total administration time is 15 to 20 minutes and requires very little training. Reliability data presented in the manual looks promising (interrater reliability = 0.98; parallel form reliability = 0.91). It is important to note that comparatively little normative data are available and little data concerning the initial standardization sample are presented in the test manual. Clinicians who wish to use this device should do so with caution initially until a clinical familiarity is achieved.

KAUFMAN SHORT NEUROPSYCHOLOGICAL ASSESSMENT PROCEDURE

The Kaufman Short Neuropsychological Assessment Procedure (K-SNAP) (American Guidance Service, Inc., personal communication, Sep-

TABLE 10.10   Item Content for the MEAMS

1.   Orientation—time and place
2.   Name Learning (visual-verbal association learning)
3.   Naming
4.   Comprehension (identify objects from description)
5.   Remembering Pictures (recognition memory)
6.   Arithmetic (simple calculation)
7.   Spatial Construction (copy two geometrical figures)
8.   Fragmented Letter Perception
9.   Unusual Views (common objects viewed from different angles)
10. Usual Views
11. Verbal Fluency
12. Motor Perseveration (based on verbal contingencies)
Scoring: 1 point for each subtest passed
           Maximum score = 12
           10–12 points   = normal performance
           8–9 points   = borderline performance
           < 8 points   = impaired performance

tember 1993; Kaufman & Kaufman, in press); is the newest entry into the screening game. Scheduled to be released in early 1994, the K-SNAP is designed to be a brief, individually administered, nationally normed measure of mental functioning at three levels of complexity: (1) a lower level of attention-orientation (essentially a Mental Status section); (2) an intermediate level of simple memory and perception skills (Number Recall and Gestalt Closure subtests); and (3) a high level of complex intellectual functioning and planning ability (Four-Letter Words subtest). The authors note that the K-SNAP is designed for use with individuals ranging in age from 11 years to over 90 years. Administration time is reported to be about 20 to 30 minutes.

The K-SNAP comes in a basic AGS easel kit that contains the four subtests, a record form containing the items for the Four-Letter Words subtest, as well as space for recording biographical information, raw scores, and derived scores. Detailed instructions and normative data are provided in the test manual.

In the Mental Status Subtest, patients are required to respond to simple questions assessing attention and orientation to the world around them. The Number Recall Subtest is a digit span–type task with number series ranging from 2 to 9 digits. In the Gestalt Closure Subtest the individuals are asked to name an object or scene pictured in a partially completed "inkblot" drawing. The final subtest Four-Letter Words, requires the patient to determine the "secret word" by studying clues presented and generating decision-making strategies.

The intermediate and high-level subtest scores are combined to yield a composite score. The two intermediate level subtests yield a Recall/Closure composite score. An Impairment Index is generated based on the application of a set of diagnostic criteria to the subtest and composite scores of the K-SNAP.

Little other information is available at the time this edition of the book was being written concerning the K-SNAP. The devices appear to be face valid and seems to have the needed components of a useful screening device. That there is normative data and reported validity and reliability data is a definite plus; however, until the instrument is made available for use the clinical utility of the test cannot be determined.

Glossary

abducens nerve—The sixth cranial nerve. Lesions here can result in excessive lacrimation.

abscess—A circumscribed infection characterized by a buildup of pus surrounded by a thick wall of cells.

absence seizures—A form of epilepsy, typically found in children, characterized by a brief altered state of consciousness (petit mal seizures).

abulia—Inability to perform voluntary acts or make decisions.

acalculia—See dyscalculia. An acquired reduction in the ability of a person to perform arithmetic calculations.

acoustic nerve—The eighth cranial nerve. It has two divisions: the cochlear division, which is partly responsible for the transmission of auditory information to the brain, and the vestibular division, which is responsible for the sense of balance.

acoustic neuroma—A tumor, largely comprised of nerve cells and nerve fibers, that often compromises function of the acoustic division of the eighth cranial nerve.

acromegaly—A chronic disease of the endocrine system resulting in elongation and enlargement of certain bone structures, including the frontal bones and jaw bones. Symptoms include muscular pain, headaches, and sweating.

Addison's disease—A condition resulting from a deficiency in secretion of adrenocortical hormones. Symptoms include anorexia, weight loss, nausea, weakness, and fatigue.

afferent fibers—Neuronal pathways that carry information upward toward the cerebral cortex from peripheral areas of the nervous system.

agnosia—Literally, a condition of not knowing. It is the inability to recognize sensory stimuli. Color agnosia is the inability to recognize colors.

Visual agnosia is the inability to recognize objects in the presence of intact visual sensation.

agrammatism—A defect in the syntactical composition of the patient's verbal output. It is characterized by the omission of most relational words, including articles, prepositions, and conjunctions.

agraphia—An acquired condition of impaired or absent writing ability.

akathisia—A condition of extreme motor restlessness. It is accompanied by subjective feelings of anxiety and restlessness.

akinesia—A state of lowered motor activity.

akinetic mutism—A state of wakeful unresponsiveness in which there is no apparent purposeful mental activity. The person appears to be awake, but inactive.

alexia—An acquired inability to read.

Alzheimer's disease—A dementia characterized by progressive mental impairment and by the presence of excessive neurofibrillary tangles and senile plaques.

amnesia—A partial or total impairment of memory functions. *Anterograde amnesia* is a disturbance of memory that follows some etiologic event. It is a disturbance of the transfer of engrams from short-term into long-term memory storage. *Retrograde amnesia* is a disturbance of memory prior to the ecologic event. It is a disturbance of retrieval from long-term storage.

amygdala—One of the structures of the limbic system, important in memory and in the regulation of emotion.

amyotrophic lateral sclerosis—A condition of muscle weakness and atrophy, with spasticity and hyperreflexia. It is the result of degeneration of motor neurons of the spinal cord, medulla, and cortex.

aneurysm—A weak wall of a vein or artery that dilates and fills with blood and that may hemorrhage, destroying surrounding neural tissue.

angular gyrus—A region of the cerebral cortex, in the area of the posterior parietal lobe, which is intimately involved in the production of speech.

anisocoria—A condition wherein the pupils dilate unevenly to light.

anomia—Sometimes known as "dysnomia," it is a condition in which the patient has difficulty finding correct words. It is often assessed by a confrontation naming task.

anosmia—Lack of the sense of smell. Although it is sometimes associated with lesions of the olfactory nerve (cranial nerve 1), it is more frequently associated with non–central nervous system dysfunction, such as peripheral disease of the nostrils.

anosognosia—A condition in which the patient is unaware of existing deficits. It occurs despite objective evidence that deficits exists and is often associated with lesions in the posterior nondominant hemisphere.

anterior cerebral artery—An artery that originates from the internal carotid artery and principally serves the frontal lobes, corpus callosum, olfactory, and optic tracts.

anterior communicating artery—An artery that originates from the anterior cerebral artery, supplies the caudate nucleus, and helps form the anterior part of the Circle of Willis.

anterograde amnesia—Loss of memory for events that follow cerebral trauma, such as often occurs in head injuries.

anticholinergic drugs—Drugs that interfere with passage of nerve impulses through the parasympathetic nerves.

Anton's syndrome—A form of anosognosia in which the patient is totally blind but lacks awareness of his blindness.

aphasia—An acquired inability to use certain aspects of language. It can be either an expressive or a receptive language disorder. "Aphasia" is a very broad term that is made more useful by descriptive qualifiers indicating the type of language impairment involved.

aphemia—Nonfluent speech with intact writing skills.

apraxia—Impaired ability to perform previously chained skills in a continuous behavior. **Construction apraxia** is an impairment in reproducing patterns; it is assessed by observing drawing and drafting or by having the patient build three-dimensional objects. **Ideational apraxia** refers to impairment in the idea of the required behavior; it is usually assessed by asking the patient to perform several linked behaviors. **Ideomotor apraxia** refers to the inability to demonstrate motor behaviors that were known in the past; it is assessed by asking the patient to pantomime a task, such as using a can opener or using a pair of scissors.

aprosody—A condition in which the coloring, rhythm, melody, cadence, intonation, or emphasis of speech is impaired. A person with this condition is likely to speak in a monotone even when relaying affective material.

Aqueduct of Sylvius—A narrow canal, about three-quarters of an inch long, that connects the third and fourth ventricles.

arachnoid—The middle layer of the meninges. The term means "like a cobweb" and is used because of the delicate nature of the arachnoid.

arachnoid space—The space around the arachnoid layer that is filled with fibrous tissue and acts as a conduit for cerebrospinal fluid.

arteriosclerosis—A disease of the vascular system characterized by cumulative buildup of fatty deposits on the inner walls of veins and arteries.

arteriovenous malformation—Abnormally shaped arteries and veins. It may be only a small tangle of vessels or a large collection of abnormal vessels occupying a large area.

astereognosis—An acquired inability to recognize an object by the sense of touch. It is assessed by handing an object to a blindfolded patient and asking the patient to identify the object.

astrocytoma—A type of neoplasm that develops from astrocyte cells. These tumors are typically unencapsulated and intracerebral.

ataxia—Loss or failure of muscular coordination. Movement, especially gait, is clumsy and appears to be uncertain. Ataxic patients often sway while walking. Ataxia usually results from an inaccurate sense of position caused by distorted proprioception in the lower limbs. Difficulty with gait increases greatly when the patient is asked to walk with eyes closed.

athetosis—A movement disorder in which involuntary undulating, or writhing movements occur. These are called "athetoid movements"; they are slower and more sustained than choreiform movements and are associated with increased muscle tone.

atonia—Complete lack of muscle tone.

atrophy—Shrinkage of (brain) tissue due to loss of neuronal processes.

attention—The capacity of an individual to screen out certain aspects of the environment and to perceive and process other aspects.

auditory nerve—Sometimes called the "vestibular" or "acoustic nerve." It is the eighth cranial nerve and transmits auditory information and also is involved in the sense of equilibrium. (See also **acoustic nerve**.)

auditory verbal dysnomia—An aphasic deficit characterized by impairment of ability to understand the symbolic significance of verbal communication through the auditory avenue (loss of auditory-verbal comprehension).

aura—A sensory phenomenon that may precede a seizure.

autoimmune disorders—Impairment of bodily processes by which immunization is effected.

autonomic nervous system—That part of the nervous system concerned with visceral and involuntary functions.

axon—The portion of a neuron that transmits energy from the cell body to the receptors of other neurons.

Babinski response—Extension (instead of flexion) of the toes on stimulation of the sole of the foot, occurring in persons with lesions of the pyramidal tract.

bacterial infection—Infection by minute, one-celled organisms, which multiply by dividing in one or more directions.

ballismus—An abrupt contraction of the extremities that makes it appear as if the person is flapping or flailing her limbs. It is most commonly seen on one side of the body, in which case it is known as **hemiballismus**. Ballismus is sometimes associated with hypotonia and chorea.

basal ganglia—A portion of the brain located within the diencephalon but below the cerebral hemispheres, including the thalamus, caudate nucleus, and lentiform nucleus.

bifurcation—Division into two branches.

bradykinesis—A motor disorder, frequently seen in Parkinson's disease, which results from rigidity of muscles and which is manifested by slow finger movements and loss of fine motor skills such as writing.

brain scan—A method of identifying focal neurological disturbances by injecting a radioisotope material into an artery and scanning the head with a Geiger counter to determine where the radioisotopes are collecting.

Broca's area—A portion of the left frontal lobe intimately involved in the production of speech.

Capgras' syndrome—A condition wherein the patient is convinced that persons in his close social environment have been replaced with imposters. It is sometimes seen with nondominant hemisphere lesions, posttraumatic encephalopathy, cerebrovascular disease, and other neurological diseases, but usually only in the early stages.

carcinoma—A malignant neoplasm (cancer) that tends to infiltrate surrounding tissue and give rise to metastases.

carotid endarterectomy—A surgical technique for cleaning the vessels carrying blood to the brain.

cataplexy—An abrupt decrease in muscle tone. The person with cataplexy feels as if he has suddenly lost control of his limb(s) and may fall if the lower limbs are involved.

cerebral anoxia—A condition in which the cells of the brain do not receive sufficient oxygen to perform their normal functions.

cerebral palsy—A general term for a large number of congenital neurological disorders. The symptoms include movement disorders, weakness, spasticity, and ataxia. Some degree of mental retardation may also be present. The cause is usually some event that occurs during or shortly after the birth process.

cerebrovascular accident—An ischemic disorder that is produced by a disruption of blood flow in the brain due to an occlusion of a portion of the vascular system from a thrombus or embolus, or from a hemorrhage.

chorea—A sudden involuntary movement that serves no apparent purpose. These movements are known as **choreiform** and are brief in duration. They are asymmetric and can often be masked by the afflicted individual unless the examiner is extremely watchful. They are associated with decreased muscle tone.

clonic movements—Spasmodic alteration of contraction and relaxation such as seen in certain forms of epilepsy.

coma—A condition of profound stupor or unconsciousness.

computerized axial tomography—A neurodiagnostic technique in which x-rays measuring densities of sections of the brain are integrated by a computer.

concussion—A form of closed-head injury resulting from a blow or violent shaking of the brain.

confabulation—A symptom of Korsakoff's syndrome in which the patient supplies ready answers to questions without regard for the truth. The patient who confabulates appears to "fill in" gaps in memory with plausible facts.

conjugate—Working in unison.

constructional apraxia—See **apraxia**.

construction dyspraxia—Difficulty in reproducing (drawing) simple geometric designs and objects. See **apraxia**.

contra lateral—Referring to the opposite side of the body or brain.

contrecoup—Damage in closed-head injury that is characterized by destruction of brain tissue opposite the site of impact because of the brain's bouncing off the walls of the cranium.

contusion—A form of closed-head injury that produces mild hemorrhaging and associated swelling.

corpus callosum—The brain structure that connects the right and left hemispheres.

cortex—The outer layer of brain tissue comprised of sulci and gyri.

cranial nerves—Twelve pairs of nerves that originate in the brain and carry sensory and motor signals to and from the periphery of the central nervous system.

cyst—A sac of fluid usually associated with an infectious disorder.

déjà vu—An experience in which new experiences seem familiar and relived. Feelings of déjà vu are common with complex partial seizures.

delirium—An acute, global impairment of cognitive functioning. Delirium is usually reversible and is most often due to metabolic disturbances of brain function.

dementia—A condition, usually chronic, of global impairment of cognition that occurs in the absence of clouded consciousness. In many cases, such as in Alzheimer's disease, the condition is progressive.

Dexamethasone Suppression Test—A test designed to measure suppression of cortisol secretion in response to the administration of dexamethasone. The test is sometimes helpful in the evaluation of endogenous depression.

diplopia—Double vision.

dysarthria—Acquired impairment in motor aspects of speech. Dysarthric speech may sound slurred or compressed. **Spastic dysarthria**, associated with pseudobulbar palsy, is low in pitch and has a raspy sound, with poor articulation. **Flaccid dysarthria**, associated with bulbar palsy, has an extremely nasal aspect to its sound. **Ataxic dysarthria** is associated with cerebellar palsy and produces deficits in articulation and prosody. **Hypokinetic dysarthria**, found with parkinsonism, results in low-volume speech and less emphasis on accented syllables; there are also articulatory initiation difficulties. **Hyperkinetic dysarthria** results in prosodic, phonation, and articulatory deficits; the loudness and accents of speech are uncontrolled. There are many disorders that present with combinations of the different types of dysarthria.

dyscalculia—An aphasic symptom characterized by impairment in the ability to appreciate the symbolic significance of numbers and to perform arithmetic calculations.

dysdiadochokinesia—The inability to perform rapid alternating movements. One clinical test for this condition is to have the patient hold out both hands and probate and supinate them as rapidly as possible.

dysFluency—A disturbance of the fluency of speech.

dysgnosia—In contrast to agnosia, dysgnosia represents a partial rather than complete loss of the symbolic significance of information reaching the brain.

dyslexia—See **alexia**.

dysnomia—See **anomia**.

dysphagia—Difficulty in swallowing.

dyspnea—Labored breathing.

dyspraxia—See **apraxia**.

dystonia—Involuntary, slow movements that tend to contort a part of the body for a period. *Dystonic movements* tend to involve large portions of the body and have a sinuous quality that, when severe, resembles writhing.

edema—Swelling of the brain following cerebral insult or injury. *Cerebral edema* results from the accumulation of fluid in intercellular tissue.

embolus—Any foreign object such as an air bubble or blood clot which becomes lodged in a vessel or artery causing an occlusion of blood flow.

encephalitis—Inflammation of the brain.

epilepsy—A condition of abnormal electrical discharges from the brain associated with a temporary alteration in behavior.

eutonia—A general, pervasive feeling of physical well-being.

extrinsic—outside of the cerebral hemisphere, usually referring to neoplasms or cerebrovascular hemorrhages that are located between the skull and brain.

facial nerve—The seventh cranial nerve. It is involved in the sense of taste and contains a few other somatic sensory afferent fibers. It is also involved in facial expression. Bell's palsy is the result of compression of the seventh cranial nerve.

fissure—Any deep fold in the cerebral cortex. Fissures define the limits of the cerebral lobes.

flaccid—Relaxed, flabby, or absent muscular tone.

functional—Having a psychiatric or psychological cause.

gait—The particular manner in which a person moves while walking.

general paresis—Tertiary syphilis, characterized by progressive dementia and a generalized paralysis.

glial cells—The connective tissue of the brain (from the Latin word for "glue").

glioma—Any neoplasm arising from glial cells.

glossopharyngeal nerve—The ninth cranial nerve, consisting largely of sensory afferent fibers. Lesions here might result in the loss of the gag reflex and the carotid sinus reflex, as well as loss of the sense of taste and loss of general sensation in the lower third of the tongue.

gyrus—A convolution on the surface of the brain.

hemianopsia—The loss of vision in one-half of a visual field.

hemiballismus—See **ballismus**.

hemispatial neglect—The failure to detect, report, or orient to one side of the field of experience. Although it is possible with either hemifield, it is more long lasting when it occurs on the left side. It is also known as "hemi-attention" or "unilateral neglect."

hemorrhage—Bleeding.

homonymous hemianopsia—The loss of vision in the same half of the visual field in both eyes.

hydrocephalus—Abnormal accumulation of cerebrospinal fluid within the cranium, producing enlarged ventricles and compression of neural tissue.

hypoglossal—The twelfth cranial nerve. It has somatic efferent fibers and serves the tongue. Lesions here will result in lower motor neuron loss and contralateral hemiplegia and ipsilateral paralysis of the tongue.

hypothalamus—A structure dorsal to the thalamus that regulates sleeping, sexual activity, eating, emotions, and other behaviors.

ictal—Related to a seizure (epileptic) episode. For example, cursing is an ictal behavior associated with some forms of temporal lobe epilepsy.

ideational apraxia—See **apraxia**.

ideomotor apraxia—Sometimes called "ideokinetic apraxia." See **apraxia.**

idiopathic—A term referring to conditions whose cause is unknown. Epilepsy can be idiopathic or secondary to a known cerebral insult.

infarct—A region of dead brain tissue associated with an occlusion of the vasculature.

interictal—The period between seizure episodes in an epileptic individual.

intrinsic—Existing within the brain itself.

ipsilateral—On the same side.

ischemia—Any local and temporary deficiency of blood.

jamais vu—An experience associated with some forms of epilepsy in which familiar surroundings and experiences seem unusual or unreal.

Kayser-Fleischer ring—A brown/green ring around the cornea. This sign is pathognomonic for Wilson's disease.

Korsakoff's syndrome—Deterioration of the brain and cognitive abilities (particularly memory) caused by chronic and severe alcohol abuse and resulting thiamine deficiency.

lesion—Any damage to bodily tissues as a result of disease or injury.

meninges—Three membranes that protect the brain and provide for venous drainage. The **dura** mater, **pia** mater, and **arachnoid** layer comprise the cerebral meninges.

meningioma—A neoplasm arising in the meninges.

meningitis—Inflammation of the meninges, especially of the pia mater and the arachnoid.

metastic neoplasm—A tumor that develops from abnormal cells that have migrated from another area of the body, most commonly from the lung or breast.

micrographia—Writing with very minute letters or only on a small portion of a page. Sometimes seen in patients with seizure disorders.

minimal brain dysfunction—A term sometimes used to refer to a constellation of loosely organized symptoms. It is usually used when the etiology of these symptoms is unknown. It has been used to describe hyperactivity, impulse control, and attention deficits, especially when it is not known for certain if the etiology is in fact organic.

motor impersistence—An inability to continue a motor activity once it is begun, despite commands to do so.

multiple sclerosis—A disease resulting from degeneration of myelin, characterized by the development of multiple plaques throughout the brain and spinal cord.

mutism—A condition of not speaking, dumbness. **(See akinetic mutism**.)

myelopathy—Disintegration of the myelin sheath. Not to be confused with myopathy.

myoclonus—An abrupt contraction of musculature. Myoclonus results in a jerking motion and ordinarily occurs when a person is falling asleep. Myoclonus in the waking stages may be indicative of neuropathology.

myopathy—Degeneration of muscle fiber. Not to be confused with myelopathy.

myotonia—Delayed relaxation of the muscles. *Myotonic dystrophy* appears in adulthood and is characterized by an inability of the patient to release a grasp or undo any motor contraction quickly.

myxedema—An endocrine disorder in which there is hypofunction of the thyroid, resulting in psychomotor slowing, apathy, and drowsiness.

neoplasm—Literally "new growth," the term refers to a tumor.

neuralgia—Acute, paroxysmal pain along the course of a nerve.

neuritis—Inflammation of a nerve.

nystagmus—A spasmodic movement of the eyes, either rotary or side to side.

oculomotor nerve—The third cranial nerve. It has efferent fibers to the eye muscles. It is responsible for accommodation and pupil dilation, among other motor activities. Lesions may result in anisocoria, ptosis, or strabismus.

olfactory nerve—The first cranial nerve, serving the sense of smell.

Optic nerve—The second cranial nerve, serving the sense of sight.

papilledema—Swelling of the optic disc.

paraphasia—A disturbance in the verbal output of a patient. A literal paraphasia involves the substitution of letters in a word, for example, "ridilicous" for "ridiculous." Semantic or verbal paraphasia involves the substitution of one word for another. The two words are usually in the same semantic class, for example "shirt" for "pants."

parathesia—Abnormalities of sensation, especially tactile and somesthetic sensation.

Parkinson's disease—A disorder that primarily affects the motor functions of the cerebellum. Parkinson's disease is characterized by tremors and gait disturbances.

pathognomonic signs—Any sign or symptom that is characteristic of a disease or pathological condition and that does not occur in the absence of pathology.

Pick's disease—A form of dementia that affects the frontal and temporal lobes and that is characterized by early loss of social grace and inhibition.

presenile dementia—Severe deterioration of mental functions before the age of 65. Most contemporary investigators minimize the utility of the distinction between presenile and senile dementias.

prosopagnosia—An acquired inability to recognize familiar faces, usually associated with bilateral posterior lesions. (It is different from an inability to recognize unfamiliar faces, which is associated with right posterior lesions.)

pseudodementia—Any form of apparent cognitive impairment that is not global and that mimics dementia. A common form is pseudodementia secondary to depression.

ptosis—Permanent dropping of the upper eyelid.

reduplicative paramnesia—A condition whereby the patient has very strong feelings that the current, novel, and unfamiliar environment is actually familiar and personally important. An extremely rare phenomenon.

rigidity—Increased muscle tone that manifests itself as resistance to passive movement.

scanning speech—Slowed speech with pauses between each syllable.

scotoma—A blind or partially blind area in the visual field.

senile dementia—Severe deterioration of mental functions in persons over the age of 65 years. See **presenile dementia.**

senile plaques—Areas of incomplete necrosis found in persons with primary neuronal degenerative diseases of the brain. Senile plaques can also be found, in the absence of overt pathology, in most elderly people.

spasm—An involuntary contraction of a muscle group. It can be associated with anxiety or fear as well as with a neurological disorder.

spasticity—Abnormal increases in muscle tone.

spinal accessory nerve—The eleventh cranial nerve. It has effluent fibers for the branchiomeric musculature. A lesion here might result in paralysis of the trapezium.

stereognosis—The ability to use tactile cues to recognize objects and shapes.

stereotypy—Repetitive movements that serve no purpose.

strabismus—Lack of muscle coordination such that both eyes cannot be directed to the same object.

stroke—A general term used to describe those disorders of the brain that are characterized by disruption of blood flow.

subdural hematoma—A lesion that results from bleeding into the subdural space.

suppression—Any failure to perceive a stimulus on one side of the body with bilateral simultaneous stimulation. Suppressions can exist with auditory, visual, or tactile stimulation. Synonym: extinction.

synapse—The space between the terminal end of an axon and another cell body. Neurotransmitters are released in the synapse and carry signals from one nerve cell to another.

tentorium—The structure that divides the cerebrum from the cerebellum.

thombus—Any blood clot that forms in an artery or vessel, creating an occlusion. The thrombus typically forms at the bifurcation of a vessel.

tic—Stereotyped movements that may be simple or complex. They are most commonly found in the muscles of the face and are sensitive to changes in the level of subjective tension.

tinnitus—Ringing in the ears.

transient ischemic attacks (TIAs)—Brief episodes of insufficient blood supply to selected portions of the brain.

tremor—An oscillatory or shaking motion.

trigeminal nerve—The fifth cranial nerve. It has afferent fibers from the face and forehead. It is the conduit for sensation of pain, tactile sensation, and thermal sensation. It also has efferent fibers for the mucous membranes, nose, mouth, teeth, and speech apparatus. It is responsible for the corneas reflex, the tearing reflex, and sneezing.

tochlear nerve—The fourth cranial nerve. It has efferent fibers innervating skeletal muscles. Vertical diplopia is one symptom of a lesion in the trochlear nerve.

unilateral neglect—See **hemispatial neglect**.

vagus—The tenth cranial nerve. It has an inhibitory effect on heart rate. It has several efferent and adherent fibers to the speech apparatus. Lesions here can result in paralysis of the soft palate, pharynx, and larynx. Possible symptoms include hoarseness, dyspnea, dysphagia, or dysarthria.

ventricles—The spaces within the brain through which cerebrospinal fluid circulates.

vertigo—A sensation of spinning or the perception that external objects are revolving around an individual. Often used somewhat imprecisely to refer to a feeling of dizziness.

vorbeireden—A verbal response that is incorrect but that indicates the patient understood the nature of the question as well as the correct answer.

Wernicke's aphasia—An acquired inability to communicate verbally due to impairment of receptive abilities. Associated with lesions in the posterior portion of the dominant hemisphere.

Wilson's disease—An autosomal recessive genetic disorder of copper metabolism; also known as hepatolenticular degeneration.

witzelsucht—Inappropriate jocularity, most commonly found with right hemisphere lesions.

References

Adams, J. (1966). *An investigation of school children on Canter's Background Interference procedure for the Bender-Gestalt*. Unpublished master's thesis, University of Iowa.

Adams, K.M., & Heaton, R. (1990). The NIMH Neuropsychological Battery. *Journal of Clinical and Experimental Neuropsychology, 12*, 960–953.

Adams, R.D., & Victor, M. (1977). *Principles of neurology*. New York: McGraw-Hill.

Adams, R.D., & Victor, M. (1981). *Principles of neurology* (2nd ed.). New York: McGraw-Hill.

Armitage, S.B. (1946). An analysis of certain psychological tests used for the evaluation of brain-injury. *Psychological Monographs, 60*.

Army Individual Test. (1944). Manual of directions and scoring. Washington, D.C.: War Department, Adjutant General's Office.

Bachman, D.L., Wolf, P.A., Linn, R., Knoefel, J.E., Cobb, J., Belanger, A., D'Agostino, & White, L.R. (1992). Prevalence of dementia of probable presenile dementia of the Alzheimer type in the Framingham study. *Neurology, 42*, 115–119.

Barona, A., Reynolds, C.R., & Chastain, R. (1984). A demographically based index of pre-morbid intelligence for the WAIS-R. *Journal of Consulting and Clinical Psychology, 52*, 885–887.

Barry, P. (1991). Unpublished Manual for the Barry Rehabilitation Inpatient Screening of Cognition. Scottsdale, AZ.

Barry, P., Clark, D.E., Yaguda, M., Higgins, G.E., & Mangel, H. (1989). Rehabilitation inpatient screening of early cognitive recovery. *Archives of Physical Medicine and Rehabilitation, 70*, 902–906.

Beaumont, J.G., & Davidoff. (1992). Assessment of visuo-perceptual dysfunction. In J.R. Crawford, D.M. Parker, & W.W. McKinlay (Eds.), *A handbook of neuropsychological assessment*. Hove, UK: Lawrence Erlbaum.

Battersby, W.S., Bender, M.B., Pollack, M., & Kahn, R.L. (1956). Unilateral "spatial agnosia" ("inattention") in patients with cortical lesions. *Brain, 35*, 68–93.

Bender, L.A. (1938). *A visual motor gestalt test and its clinical use* (American Orthopsychiatric Association Research Monographs No. 3).

Benton, A.L. (1967). Problems in test construction in the field of aphasia. *Cortex, 3*, 32–58.

Benton, A.L. (1968). Differential behavioral effects in frontal lobe disease. *Neuropsychologia, 6*, 53–60.

Benton, A.L. (1973). The measurement of aphasic disorders. In A.C. Velasquez (Ed.), *Aspectos patologicos del lengage* (pp. 141–192). Lima: Centro Neuropsicologico.

Benton, A.L. (1974). *The Revised Visual Retention Test* (4th ed.). New York: Psychological Corporation.

Benton, A.L., Elithorn, A., Fogel, M.L., & Kerr, M.A. (1963). A perceptual maze test sensitive to brain damage. *Journal of Neurology, Neurosurgery, and Psychiatry, 26*, 540–543.

Benton, A.L., Eslinger, R., & Damasio, K. (1981). Normative observations on neuropsychological test performance in old age. *Journal of Clinical Neuropsychology, 3*, 35–42.

Benton, A.L., Hamsher, K. deS., Varney, N.R., & Spreen, O. (1983). *Contributions to neuropsychological assessment*. New York: Oxford University Press.

Benton, A.L., & Van Allen, M.W. (1968). Impairment in facial recognition in patients with cerebral disease. *Cortex, 4*, 344–358.

Benton, A.L., & Van Allen, M.W. (1972). Aspects of neuropsychological assessment in patients with cerebral disease. In C.M. Geitz (Ed.), *Aging and the brain* (pp. 246–285). New York: Plenum.

Benton, A.L., Van Allen, M.W., & Fogel, M.L. (1964). Temporal orientation in cerebral disease. *Journal of Nervous and Mental Disease, 139*, 110–119.

Berg, E.A. (1948). A simple objective technique for measuring flexibility in thinking. *Journal of General Psychology, 39*, 15–22.

Billingslea, F.Y. (1965). The Bender-Gestalt: A review and a perspective. *Psychological Bulletin, 60*, 233–251.

Black, F.W. (1974). The cognitive sequelae of penetrating missile wounds of the brain. *Military Medicine, 139*, 815–820.

Blair, J.R., & Spreen, O. (1989). Predicting premorbid IQ: A revision of the National Adult Reading Test. *The Clinical Neuropsychologist, 3*, 129–136.

Boll, T.J., & Reitan, R.M. (1975). Effect of age on performance on the Trail Making Test. *Perceptual and Motor Skills, 36*, 691–694.

Boller, F., & Vignolo, L.A. (1966). Latent sensory aphasia in hemisphere-damaged patients: An experimental study with the Token Test. *Brain, 89*, 815–831.

Bond, M.R. (1986). Neurobehavioral sequelae of closed head injury. In 1. Grant & K.M. Adams (Eds.), *Neuropsychological assessment of neuropsychiatric disorders* (pp. 347–373). New York: Oxford University Press.

Bornstein, R.A., & Chelune, G. J. (1988). Factor structure of the Wechsler Memory Scale-Revised. *The Clinical Neuropsychologist, 2*, 107–114.

Borowski, J.G., Benton, A.L., & Spreen, O. (1967). Word fluency and brain damage. *Neuropsychologia, 5*, 135–140.

Brilliant, P.J., & Gynther, M.D. (1963). Relationships between performance on three tests for organicity and selected patient variables. *Journal of Consulting Psychology, 27*, 474–479.

Brown, G.G., Baird, S.D., & Shatz, M.W. (1986). The effects of vascular disease and its treatment on higher cortical functioning. In 1. Grant & K.M. Adams (Eds.), *Neuropsychological assessment of neuropsychiatric disorders* (pp. 384–414). New York: Oxford University Press.

Bubb, D.I. (1984). *Neurologic problems*. Oradell, NJ: Medical Economics Books.

Buschke, H. (1973). Selective reminding for analysis of memory and learning. *Journal of Verbal Learning and Verbal Behavior, 12*, 543–550.

Buschke, H., & Fuld, P.A. (1974). Evaluating storage, retention, and retrieval in disordered memory and learning. *Neurology, 24*, 1019–1025.

Butters, N., & Barton, M. (1970). Effect of parietal lobe damage on the performance of reversible operations in space. *Neuropsychologia, 8*, 205–214.

Butters, N., Grant, I., Haxby, J., Judd, L.L., Martin, A., McClelland, J., Pequegnat, W., Schacter, D., & Stover, E. (1990). Assessment of AIDS-related cognitive changes: Recommendations of the NIMH Workgroup on neuropsychological assessment approaches. *Journal of Clinical and Experimental Neuropsychology, 12*, 963–978.

Caine, E.D. (1986). The neuropsychology of depression: The pseudodementia syndrome. In I Grant & K.M. Adams (Eds.), *Neuropsychological assessment of neuropsychiatric disorders* (pp. 221–243). New York: Oxford University Press.

Canter, A. (1966). A background interference procedure to increase sensitivity of the Bender-Gestalt Test to organic brain damage. *Journal of Consulting Psychology, 30*, 91–95.

Canter, A. (1971). A comparison of the background interference procedure effect in schizophrenic, nonschizophrenic and organic patients. *Journal of Clinical Psychology, 27*, 473–477.

Canter, A. (1976). *The Canter Background Interference Procedure for the Bender-Gestalt Test*. Nashville: Counselor Recordings.

Chelune, G.J., & Baer, R.A. (1986). Developmental norms for the Wisconsin Card Sorting test. *Journal of Clinical and Experimental Neuropsychology, 8*, 219–228.

Chelune, G.J., & Bornstein, R.A. (1988). WMS-R patterns among patients with unilateral brain lesions. *The Clinical Neuropsychologist, 2*, 121–132.

Chouinard, M.-J., & Braun, C.M.J. (1993). A meta-analysis of the relative sensitivity of neuropsychological screening tests. *Journal of Clinical and Experimental Neuropsychology, 15*, 591–607.

Cimino, C., Behner, G., Cattarin, J., & Tantleff, S. (1991, February). *Construct validity of the "Assessment of Cognitive Skills" (ACS)*. Paper presented at the annual North American meeting of the International Neuropsychological Society, San Diego.

Colonna, A., & Faglioni, R (1966). The performance of hemisphere-damaged patients on spatial intelligence tests. *Cortex, 2*, 293–307.

Costa, L.D. (1975). The relation of visuospatial dysfunction to digit span performance in patients with cerebral lesions. *Cortex, 11*, 31–36.

Costa, L.D., Vaughan, H.G., Levita, E., & Farber, N. (1963). Purdue Pegboard as a predictor of the presence and laterality of cerebral lesions. *Journal of Consulting Psychology, 27*, 133–137.

Costello, S.D., Bieliauskas, L.A., & Terpenning, M. (1992, August). *The sensitivity of neuropsychological screening instruments: A comparison of the*

MMSE and the NCSE. Paper presented at the annual meeting of the American Psychological Association, Washington, D.C.

Crawford, J.R. (1992). Current and premorbid intelligence measures in neuropsychological assessment. In J.R. Crawford, D.M. Parker, & W.W. McKinlay (Eds.), *A handbook of neuropsychological assessment*. East Sussex, United Kingdom: Lawrence Erlbaum.

Crow, R.R. (1982) Recent genetic research in schizophrenia. In F.A. Henn & H.A. Nasrallah (Eds.), *Schizophrenia as a brain disease* (pp. 40–55). New York: Oxford University Press.

Cummings, J.L. (1985). *Clinical neuropsychiatry*. Orlando, FL: Grune & Stratton.

Dal Canto, M.C. (1989). AIDS and the nervous system. *Human Pathology, 20*, 410–416.

Davies, A. (1968). The influence of age on Trail Making Test performance. *Journal of Clinical Psychology, 24*, 96–98.

DeRenzi, E. (1968). Nonverbal memory and hemispheric side of lesion. *Neuropsychologia, 6*, 181–189.

DeRenzi, E., Faglioni, P., Savoiardo, M., & Vignolo, L.A. (1966). The influence of aphasia and of the hemisphere side of the cerebral lesion on abstract thinking. *Cortex, 2*, 399–420.

DeRenzi, E., Pieczuro, A., & Vignolo, L.A. (1968). Ideational apraxia: A quantitative study. *Neuropsychologia, 6*, 41–52.

De Renzi, E., & Spinnler, H. (1967). Visual recognition in patients with unilateral cerebral disease. *Journal of Nervous and Mental Disease, 142*, 515–525.

DeRenzi, E., & Vignolo, L.A. (1962). The Token Test: A sensitive test to detect disturbances in aphasics. *Brain, 85*, 665–678.

Diller, L., Ben-Yishay, Y., Gerstman, L.J., Goodkin, R., Gordon, W., & Weinberg, J. (1974). *Studies in cognition and rehabilitation in hemiplegia* (Research Monograph No. 50). New York: New York University Medical Center, Institute of Rehabilitation Medicine.

Dodrill, C.B. (1978). The hand dynamometer as a neuropsychological measure. *Journal of Consulting and Clinical Psychology, 46*, 1432–1435.

Duffy, F.H. (1981). Brain electrical activity mapping (BEAM): Computerized access to complex brain function. *International Journal of Neuroscience, 13*, 55–65.

Duffy, F.H. (1982). Topographic display of evoked potentials: Clinical applications of brain electrical activity mapping (BEAM). *Annals of the New York Academy of Science, 388*, 183–196.

Duffy, F.H., Albert, M.S., & McAnulty, G. (1984). Brain electrical activity in patients with presenile and senile dementia of the Alzheimer's type. *Annals of Neurology, 16*, 439–448.

Dunn, L.M., & Dunn, L.M. (1981). *Peabody Picture Vocabulary Test-Revised*. Circle Pines, MN: American Guidance Service.

Dunn, L.M., & Markwardt, F.C. (1970). *Peabody Individual Achievement Test*. Circle Pines, MN: American Guidance Service.

Dvorine, I. (1953). *Dvorine Pseudo-Isochromatic Plates* (2nd ed.). Baltimore: Waverly Press.

Eisenson, J. (1954). *Examining for aphasia: A manual for the examination of aphasia and related disturbances.* New York: Psychological Corporation.

Eisenson, J. (1973). *Adult aphasia.* New York: Appleton-Century-Crofts.

Ekstrom, R.B., French, J.W., Harman, H.H., & Dermen, D. (1976). *Manual for Kit of Factor-Referenced Cognitive Tests.* Princeton, New Jersey: Education Testing Service.

Elithorn, A. (1955). A preliminary report on a perceptual maze test sensitive to brain damage. *Journal of Neurology, Neurosurgery, and Psychiatry, 18,* 287–289.

Erickson, R.C., Calsyn, D.A., & Scheupbach, C.S. (1978). Abbreviating the Halstead-Reitan Neuropsychological Test Battery. *Journal of Clinical Psychology, 34,* 922–926.

Evans, D.A. (1990). Estimated prevalence of Alzheimer's disease in the United States. *Milbank Quarterly, 68,* 267–289.

Feldman, R.G., Ricks, N. L., & Baker, E.L. (1980). Neuropsychological effects of industrial toxins: A review. *American Journal of Industrial Medicine, I,* 211–227.

Fields, R.B., Starratt, C., Fishman, E., Cisewski, D., & Coffey, C.E. (1993). Detecting change in cognitive status following treatment for organic mood disorder: MMSE vs. NCSE. In National Academy of Neuropsychology: Abstracts from the 12th annual meeting, Pittsburgh, PA, November 5–7, 1992. *Archives of Clinical Neuropsychology, 8,* 223.

Flor-Henry, P. (1976). Lateralized temporal-limbic dysfunction and psychopathology. *Annals of the New York Academy of Science, 286,* 779–795.

Fogel, M.L. (1965). The Proverbs Test in the appraisal of cerebral disease. *Journal of General Psychology, 72,* 269–275.

Folstein, M.E., Folstein, S.E., & McHugh, P.R. (1975). ''Mini-Mental State'': A practical method for grading the cognitive state of patients for the clinician. *Journal of Psychiatric Research, 12,* 189–198.

Friedland, R.P., Budinger, T.F., Brant-Zawadzki, M., & Jagust, W.J. (1984). The diagnosis of Alzheimer-type dementia. *Journal of the American Medical Association, 252,* 2750–2752.

Garron, D.C., & Cheifetz, D.I. (1965). Comment on ''Bender Gestalt discernment of organic pathology.'' *Psychological Bulletin, 63,* 197–200.

Gates, A.I., & MacGinitie, W.H. (1969). *Gates-MacGinitie Reading Tests.* New York: Teachers College Press.

Geffen, G., Hoar, K.J., O'Hanlon, A.P., Clark, C.R., & Geffen, L.B. (1990). Performance measures of 16- to 86-year-old males and females on the Auditory Verbal Learning Test. *Clinical Neuropsychologist, 4,* 45–63.

Glenner, G. (1982). Alzheimer's disease (senile dementia): A research update and critique with recommendations. *Journal of the American Geriatric Society, 30,* 59–62.

Gold, J.M., Randolph, C., Carpenter, C.J., Goldberg, T.E., & Weinberger, D.R. (1992). Performance of patients with schizophrenia in the Wechsler Memory Scale-Revised. *The Clinical Neuropsychologist, 6,* 367–373.

Golden, C.J. (1975). A group version of the Stroop Color and Word Test. *Journal of Personality Assessment, 39,* 386–391.

Golden, C.J. (1976). The identification of brain damage by an abbreviated form of the Halstead-Reitan Neuropsychological Battery. *Journal of Clinical Psychology, 32*, 821–826.

Golden, C.J. (1977a). The validity of the Halstead-Reitan neuropsychological battery in a mixed psychiatric and brain damaged population. *Journal of Consulting and Clinical Psychology, 45*, 1043–1048.

Golden, C.J. (1977b). Identification of brain disorders by the Stroop and Word Test. *Journal of Clinical Psychology, 32*, 621–626.

Golden, C.J. (1977c). The identification of brain damage by an abbreviated form of the Halstead-Reitan Neuropsychological Battery. *Journal of Clinical Psychology, 32*, 821–828.

Golden, C.J. (1978). *The Stroop Color and Word Test: A manual for clinical and experimental uses*. Chicago: Stoelting.

Golden, C.J. (1979). *Clinical interpretation of objective psychological tests*. New York: Grune & Stratton.

Golden, C.J. (1981). *Diagnosis and rehabilitation in clinical neuropsychology* (2nd ed.). Springfield, IL: Charles C. Thomas.

Golden, C.J., Hammeke, T.A., & Purisch, A.D. (1985). *The Luria-Nebraska Neuropsychological Battery*. Los Angeles: Western Psychological Services.

Golden, C.J., Moses, J.A., Coffman, J.A., Miller, W.R., & Strider, F.D. (1983). *Clinical Neuropsychology: Interface with neurologic and psychiatric disorders*. New York: Grune & Stratton.

Golden, C.J., Osmon, D.C., Moses, J.A., Jr., & Berg, R.A. (1981). *Interpretation of the Halstead-Reitan Neuropsychological Battery: A casebook approach*. New York: Grune & Stratton.

Golding, E. (1989). *The Middlesex Elderly Assessment of Mental State*. Fareham, UK: Thames Valley Test Company.

Goldstein, G. (1986). The neuropsychology of schizophrenia. In I. Grant & K.M. Adams (Eds.), *Neuropsychological assessment of neuropsychiatric disorders* (pp. 147–171). New York: Oxford University Press.

Goldstein, K.H., & Scheerer, M. (1948). *Abstract and concrete behavior: An experimental study with special tests. Psychological Monographs, 53*, Whole No. 239.

Goldstein, K.H., & Scheerer, M. (1953). Tests of abstract and concrete behavior. In A. Weider (Ed.), *Contributions to medical psychology* (Vol. 2, pp. 124–172). New York: Ronald Press.

Gollin, E.S. (1960). Developmental studies of visual recognition of incomplete objects. *Perceptual and Motor Skills, 11*, 289–298.

Gorham, D.R. (1956). A Proverbs Test for clinical and experimental use. *Psychological Reports, 2*, (Suppl. 1) 1–12.

Graham, F.K., & Kendall, B.S. (1960). Memory-for-Designs Test: Revised general manual. *Perceptual and Motor Skills, 11*, (Suppl. 2–VII) 147–188.

Grant, D.A., & Berg, E.A. (1948). A behavioral analysis of degree of reinforcement and ease of shifting to new responses in a Weigl-type card-sorting problem. *Journal of Experimental Psychology, 38*, 401–411.

Grant, I., & Adams, K.M. (Eds.). (1986). *Neuropsychological assessment of neuropsychiatric disorders*. New York: Oxford University Press.

Guertin, W.H., Ladd, C.E., Frank, G.H., Rabin, A.L., & Hiester, D.S. (1966). Research with the Wechsler Intelligence Scales for Adults: 1960–1965. *Psychological Bulletin, 66*, 385–409.

Hain, J.D. (1964). The Bender-Gestalt Test: A scoring method for identifying brain damage. *Journal of Consulting Psychology, 28*, 34–40.

Hall, R.C.W. (1980). Depression. In R.C.W. Hall (Ed.), *Psychiatric presentations of medical illness: Somatopsychic disorders* (pp. 37–63). New York: SP Medical & Scientific Books.

Halstead, W.C. (1947). *Brain and intelligence*. Chicago: University of Chicago Press.

Halstead, W.C., & Wepman, J.M. (1959). The Halstead-Wepman Aphasia Screening Test. *Journal of Speech and Hearing Disorders, 14*, 9–15.

Hannay, J.H. (1986). *Experimental techniques in human neuropsychology*. New York: Oxford University Press.

Hannay, J.H., & Levin, H.S. (1985). Selective Reminding Test: An examination of the equivalence of four forms. *Journal of Clinical and Experimental Neuropsychology, 7*, 251–263.

Hartje, W., Kerschensteiner, M., Poeck, K., & Argass, B. (1973). A cross-validation study on the Token Test. *Neuropsychologia, 11*, 119–121.

Hartley, L.L. (1990). Assessment of functional communication. In D.E. Tupper & K.D. Cicerone (Eds.), *The neuropsychology of everyday life: Assessment and basic competencies*. Boston: Kluwer Academic Publishers.

Hathaway, S.R., & McKinley, J.C. (1967). *Minnesota Multiphasic Personality Inventory*. New York: Psychological Corporation.

Heaton, R.K. (1981). *Manual for the Wisconsin Card Sorting Test*. Odessa, FL: Psychological Assessment Resources.

Heilman, K.M., & Valenstein, E. (Eds.). (1985). *Clinical neuropsychology* (2nd ed.). New York: Oxford University Press.

Heilman, K.M., Watson, R.T., & Greer, M. (1977). *Handbook for differential diagnosis of neurologic signs and symptoms*. New York: Appleton-Century Crofts.

Heimburger, R.F., & Reitan, R.M. (1961). Easily administered written test for lateralizing brain lesions. *Journal of Neurosurgery, 18*, 301–312.

Henn, F.A., & Nasrallah, H.A. (1982). *Schizophrenia as a brain disease*. New York: Oxford University Press.

Ho, D., Bredesen, D.E., Vinters, H.V., & Daar, E.S. (1989). AIDS dementia complex. *Annals of Internal Medicine, 11*, 400–409.

Horton, A.M., Jr., & Wedding, D. (1984). *Clinical and behavioral neuropsychology*. New York: Praeger.

Hulicka, I.M. (1966). Age differences in Wechsler Memory Scale scores. *Journal of Genetic Psychology, 109*, 135–145.

Hutt, M. (1969). *The Hutt adaptation of the Bender-Gestalt Test* (2nd ed.). New York: Grune & Stratton.

Isaacs, B., & Kennie, A.T. (1973). The Set Test as an aid to the detection of dementia in old people. *British Journal of Psychiatry, 123*, 467–470.

Ishihara, S. (1964). *Tests for color blindness* (11th ed.). Tokyo: Kanehara Shuppan.

Ivison, D.J. (1988). The Wechsler memory Scale: Relations between Form I and II. *Australian Psychologist, 23*, 219–224.

Jacobs, J.W., Bernhard, M.R., Delgado, A., & Strain, J.J. (1977). Screening for organic mental syndromes in the medically ill. *Annals of Internal Medicine, 86*, 40–46.

Jastak, S., & Wilkinson, G.S. (1984). *Wide Range Achievement Test*. Wilmington, DE: Jastak Associates.

Johnson, J.E., Hellkamp, D.T., & Lottman, T.J. (1971). The relationship between intelligence, brain damage, and Hutt-Briskin errors on the Bender-Gestalt. *Journal of Clinical Psychology, 27*, 84–88.

Kaemingk, K.L., & Kazniak, A.W. (1989). Neuropsychological aspects of human immunodeficiency virus infection. *The Clinical Neuropsychologist, 3*, 309–326.

Kaplan, E., Fein, D., Morris, R., & Delis, D.C. (1991). WAIS-R as a Neuropsychological Instrument. San Antonio: The Psychological Corporation.

Kaplan, E., Goodglass, H., & Weintraub, S. (1983). *Boston Naming Test*. Philadelphia, Lea & Febiger.

Kaszniak, A.W. (1986). The neuropsychology of dementia. In 1. Grant & K.M. Adams (Eds.), *Neuropsychological assessment of neuropsychiatric disorders* (pp. 172–220). New York: Oxford University Press.

Kaufman, A., and Kaufman, N. (in press). *Kaufman Short Neuropsychological Procedure*. Circle Pines, MN; American Guidance Service.

Kiernan, R.J., Mueller, J., Langston, J.W., & van Dyke, C. (1987). The Neurobehavioral Cognitive Status Examination: A brief but differentiated approach to assessment. *Annals of Internal Medicine, 107*, 481–485.

Kilpatrick, B., & Hall, R. (1980). Seizure disorders. In C.W. Hall (Ed.), *Psychiatric presentations of medical illness* (pp. 243–258). New York: Spectrum Publications.

Kimura, D. (1963). Right temporal lobe damage. *Archives of Neurology, 8*, 264–270.

Kinsbourne, M., & Warrington, E.K. (1962). A study of finger agnosia. *Brain, 85*, 47–66.

Knehr, C.A. (1965). Revised approach to detection of cerebral damage: Progressive Matrices revisited. *Psychological Reports, 17*, 71–77.

Knight, J.A., Pimental, P.A., Miller, S., & McWilliams, J. (1990, August). *Use of the Mini-Inventory of Right Brain Injury (MIRBI) in psychiatric samples*. Paper presented at the annual meeting of the American Psychological Association, Boston.

Lechtenberg, R. (1982). *The psychiatrist's guide to diseases of the nervous system*. New York: John Wiley & Sons.

Levin, H.S., & Benton, A.L. (1975). Temporal orientation in patients with brain disease. *Applied Neurophysiology, 38*, 56–60.

Levin, H.S., O'Donnell, V.M., & Grossman, R.G. (1979). The Galveston Orientation and Amnesia Test: A practical scale to assess cognition after head injury. *Journal of Nervous and Mental Disease, 167*, 675–684.

Levine, J., & Feirstein, A. (1972). Differences in test performance between brain damaged, schizophrenic, and medical patients. *Journal of Consulting and Clinical Psychology, 39*, 508–520.

Lezak, M.D. (1975, April). *When right is wrong: Vicissitudes of patients with right hemisphere lesions*. Paper presented at biennial spring meeting of the Oregon and Washington Psychological Association, Salishan, OR.

Lezak, M.D. (1976). *Neuropsychological assessment*. New York: Oxford University Press.

Lezak, M.D. (1983). *Neuropsychological assessment* (2nd ed.). New York: Oxford University Press.

Lishman, W.A. (1978). *Organic psychiatry: The psychological consequences of cerebral disorder*. London: Blackwell Scientific Publications.

Loberg, T. (1986). Neuropsychological findings in the early and middle phases of alcoholism. In I. Grant & K.M. Adams (Eds.), *Neuropsychological assessment of neuropsychiatric disorders* (pp. 415–440). New York: Oxford University Press.

Loring, D.W. (1990). The Wechsler Memory Scale-Revised or the Wechsler Memory Scale-Revisited? *The Clinical Neuropsychologist, 3,* 59–69.

Mahan, H. (1976). *Sensitivity of WAIS tests to focal lobe damage*. Unpublished manuscript.

Maj, M. (1990). Psychiatric aspects of HIV-1 infection and AIDS. *Psychological Medicine, 20,* 547–563.

Manual for the Neurobehavioral Cognitive Status Examination. (1988). Fairfax, CA: The Northern Neurobehavioral Group.

Manual for the Wechsler Individual Achievement Test. (1992). San Antonio, TX: The Psychological Corporation.

Markwardt, F.C., Jr. (1989). *Peabody Individual Achievement Test-Revised (PIAT-R) Manual*. Circle Pines, MN: American Guidance Service.

Martin, E.M., Robertson, L.C., Edelstein, H.E., Jagust, W.J., Sorenson, D.J., San-Giovanni, D., Chirirgi, V.A. (1992). Performance of patients with early HIV-1 infection on the Stroop task. *Journal of Clinical and Experimental Neuropsychology, 14,* 857–868.

Mattis, S. (1976). Mental status examination for organic mental syndrome in the elderly patient. In L. Bellak & T.B. Karasu (Eds.), *Geriatric psychiatric*. New York: Grune & Stratton.

Mattis, S.N. (1988). *Dementia rating scale*. Odessa, FL: Psychological Assessment Resources.

McFie, J. (1960). Psychological testing in clinical neurology. *Journal of Nervous and Mental Disease, 131,* 383–393.

McFie, J. (1975). *Assessment of organic intellectual impairment*. New York: Academic Press.

McManis, D.M. (1974). Memory for Designs performance of brain damaged and non-brain damaged psychiatric patients. *Perceptual and Motor Skills, 38,* 47–50.

McNamara, K.M., Wechsler, F.S., & Munger, M.P. (1984, August). *The Halstead-Reitan versus an abbreviated battery: Feasibility and Imitations*. Paper presented at the annual convention of the American Psychological Association, Toronto, Ontario, Canada.

Meier, M.J., & French, L.A. (1966). Longitudinal assessment of intellectual function following unilateral temporal lobectomy. *Journal of Clinical Psychology, 22,* 22–27.

Milner, B. (1967). Brain mechanisms suggested by studies of temporal lobes. In C.H. Millikan & F.L. Darley (Eds.). *Brain mechanisms underlying speech and language* (pp. 25–47). New York: Grune & Stratton.

Milner, B. (1962). Laterality effects in audition. In V.B. Mountcastle (Ed.), *Interhemispheric relations and cerebral dominance* (pp. 143–169). Baltimore: Johns Hopkins University Press.

Mooney, C.M., & Gerguson, G.A. (1951). A new closure test. *Canadian Journal of Psychology, 5*, 129–133.

Moran, E.J. (1990, December 5). *Hospitals,* 54.

Mortimer, J.A., & Schuman, L.M. (Eds.). (1981). *The epidemiology of dementia.* New York: Oxford University Press.

Mosher, D.L., & Smith, J.P. (1965). The usefulness of two scoring systems for the Bender Gestalt Test for identifying brain damage. *Journal of Consulting Psychology, 29*, 530–541.

Mueller, J., Kiernan, R.J., & Langston, J.W. (1988). The mental status examination. In H.H. Goldman (Ed.), *Review of general psychiatry.* Norwalk, CT: Appleton & Lange.

Nasrallah, H.A., & Weinberger, R. (1986). *The neurology of schizophrenia.* New York: Elsevier Publishing.

Natelson, B.H., Haupt, E.J., Fleisher, E.J., & Grey, L. (1979). Temporal orientation and education: A direct relationship in normal people. *Archives of Neurology, 36*, 444–446.

Navia, B.A., Jordan, B.D., & Price, R.W. (1986). The AIDS dementia complex I: Clinical features. *Annals of Neurology, 44*, 65–69.

Nehemkis, A.M., & Lewinsohn, P.M. (1972). Effects of left and right cerebral lesions in the naming process. *Perceptual and Motor Skills, 35*, 737–798.

Nelson, H.E. (1982). *National Adult Reading Test (NART): Test Manual.* Windsor, United Kingdom: NFER Nelson.

Newcombe, F. (1969). *Missile wounds of the brain.* New York: Oxford University Press.

Noble. C.E. (1961). Measurements of association value (a), rated associations (al), and scaled meaningfulness (ml) for 2100 CVC combinations of the English alphabet. *Psychological Reports, 8*, 487–521.

O'Donoghue, J.L. (1985). *Neurotoxicity of industrial and commercial chemicals* (Vols. I–II). Boca Raton, FL: CRC Press.

Olson, W.H., Brumback, R.A., Gascon, G., & Christoferson, L.A. (1981). *Practical neurology for the primary care physician.* Springfield, IL: Charles C. Thomas.

Osterrieth, P.A. (1944). La test de copie d'une figure complexes *Archives de Psychologie, 30*, 206–356.

Pajeau, A.K., & Roman, G. (1992). HIV encephalopathy and dementia. *Psychiatric Clinics of North America, 15*, 455–466.

Parsons, M. (1983). *Color atlas of clinical neurology.* Chicago: Year Book Medical Publishers.

Parsons, O.A. (1975). Brain damage in alcoholics: Altered states of unconsciousness. In M.M. Gross (Ed.), *Alcohol intoxication and withdrawal* (pp. 569–584). New York: Plenum Press.

Pascal, G.R., & Suttell, B.J. (1951). *The Bender-Gestalt Test: Quantification and validity for adults.* New York: Grune & Stratton.

Peck, D.F. (1970). The conversion of Progressive Matrices and Mill Hill vocabulary raw scores into deviation IQ's. *Journal of Clinical Psychology, 26*, 67–70.

Pimental, P., & Kingsbury, W. (1991). *Mini Inventory of Right Brain Injury (MIRBI).* Austin, TX: Pro-Ed Publishers.

Pimental, P., & Knight, J.A. (1991, October). *A cross validation study of the*

Mini-Inventory of Right Brain Injury (MIRBI). Paper presented at the annual meeting of the National Academy of Neuropsychology, Dallas.

Pincus, J.H., & Tucker, G.J. (1985). *Behavioral neurology* (3rd ed.). New York: Oxford University Press.

Porch, B.E. (1971). Multidimensional scoring in aphasia tests. *Journal of Speech and Hearing Research, 14*, 776–792.

Purdue Research Foundation. (1948). *Examiner's manual for the Purdue Pegboard*. Chicago: Science Research Associates.

Quattlebaum, L.F. (1968). A brief note on the relationship between two psychomotor tests. *Journal of Clinical Psychology, 24*, 198–199.

Raven, J.C. (1960). *Guide to the Standard Progressive Matrices*. London: H.K. Lewis.

Reddon, J.R., Gill, D.M., Gauk, S.E., & Maerz, M.D. (1988). Purdue Pegboard: Test-retest estimates. *Perceptual and Motor Skills, 66*, 503–506.

Redmond, R., & Wilson, R. (1990). *Journal of the American Optometric Association, 61*, 760–766.

Reitan, R.M. (undated). *Instructions and procedures for administering the Neuropsychological Test Battery used at the Neuropsychology Laboratory, Indiana, University Medical Center*. Unpublished manuscript.

Reitan, R.M. (1958). Validity of the Trail Making Test as an indicator of organic brain damage. *Perceptual and Motor Skills, 8*, 271–276.

Reitan, R.M. (1964). Psychological deficits resulting from cerebral lesions in man. In J.M. Warren & K. Akert (Eds.), *The frontal granular cortex and behavior* (pp. 287–306). New York: McGraw-Hill.

Reitan, R.M., & Davison, L.A. (1974). *Clinical neuropsychology: Current status and applications*. Washington DC: Winston/Wiley.

Reitan, R.M., & Wolfson, D. (1985). *The Halstead-Reitan Neuropsychological Test Battery: Theory and clinical interpretation*. Tucson, AZ: Neuropsychology Press.

Rey, A. (1941). L'examen psychologique dans les cas d'encephalopathie traumatique. *Archives de Psychologie, 28*, 286–340.

Rey, A. (1964). *L'examen clinique en psychologie* (English chapter summaries). Paris: Presses Universitaires de France.

Reynolds, C.R., & Gutkin, T.B. (1979). Predicting the premorbid intellectual status of children using demographic data. *Clinical Neuropsychology, 1*, 36–38.

Ron, M.A., Toone, B.K., & Garrelda, M.E. (1979). Diagnostic accuracy in presenile dementia. *British Journal of Psychiatry, 134*, 161–168.

Rosselli, M., & Ardila, A. (1991). Effects of age, education, and gender on the Rey-Osterreith Complex Figure. *The Clinical Neuropsychologist, 5*, 370–376.

Roth, D.L., Conboy, T.J., Reeder, K.P., & Boll, T.J. (1990). Confirmatory factor analysis of the Wechsler Memory Scale-Revised in a sample of head-injured patients. *Journal of Clinical and Experimental Neuropsychology, 12*, 834–832.

Russell, E.W. (1975). A multiple scoring method for the assessment of complex memory functions. *Journal of Consulting and Clinical Psychology, 43*, 800–809.

Russell, E.W., Neuringer, C., & Goldstein, G. (1970). *Assessment of brain dam-

age: A neuropsychological key approach. New York: John Wiley Interscience.

Sarbin, T.D. (1987). AIDS: The new "great imitator." *Journal of the American Geriatrics Society, 35*, 467–471.

Scharnhorst, S. (1992). AIDS dementia complex in the elderly: Diagnosis and management. *Nurse Practitioner, 17*, 41–43.

Schultz, E.E., Keesler, T.Y., Friedenberg, L., & Sciara, A.D. (1984). Limitations in the equivalence of alternate subtests for Russell's revision of the Wechsler Memory Scale: Causes and solutions. *Journal of Clinical Neuropsychology, 6*, 220–223.

Schwamm, van Dyke, C., Kiernan, R.J., Merrin, E.L., & Mueller, J. (1987). The Neurobehavioral Cognitive Status Examination: Comparison with the cognitive capacity screening examination and the mini-mental state examination in a neurosurgical population. *Annals of Internal Medicine, 107*, 486–491.

Seashore, C.E., Lewis, D., & Saetveit, D.L. (1960). *Seashore measures of musical talents* (rev. ed.). New York: Psychological Corporation.

Shearn, C.R., Berry, D.F., & Fitzgibbons, B. (1974). Usefulness of the Memory for Designs Test in assessing mild organic conditions in psychiatric patients. *Perceptual and Motor Skills, 38*, 1009–1015.

Sherrill, R.E. (1985). Comparison of three short forms of the Category Test. *Journal of Clinical and Experimental Neuropsychology, 7*, 231–238.

Sherrill, R.E. (1987). Options for shortening Halstead's Category Test for adults. *Archives of Clinical Neuropsychology, 2*, 343–352.

Shipley, W.C. (1967). *Manual: Shipley-Institute of Living Scale*. Los Angeles: Western Psychological Services.

Sivan, A.B. (1991). *Benton Visual Retention Test* (5th ed.). San Antonio, TX: The Psychological Corporation.

Snow, R.B., Zimmerman, R.D., Gandy, S.E., & Deck, M.D.F., (1986). Comparison of magnetic resonance imaging and computed tomography in the evaluation of head injury. *Neurosurgery, 18*, 45–52.

Song, A.Y., & Song, R.H. (1969). The Bender-Gestalt Test with background interference procedure in mental retardates. *Journal of Clinical Psychology, 25*, 69–73.

Spreen O., & Strauss, E. (1991). *A compendium of neuropsychological tests: Administration, norms, and commentary*. New York: Oxford University Press.

Starrat, C., Fields, R.B., & Cisewski, D. (1992, November). *An update on the validity of the MMSE*. Paper presented at the annual meeting of the National Academy of Neuropsychology, Pittsburgh.

Stebbins, G.T., Wilson, R.S., Gilley, D.W., Bernard, B.A., & Fox, J.H. (1990). Use of the National Adult reading Test to estimate premorbid IQ in dementia. *The Clinical Neuropsychologist, 4*, 18–24.

Street, R.F., (1931). *A Gestalt completion test*. Contributions to Education, No. 481. New York: Bureau of Publications, Teachers College, Columbia University.

Stroop, J.R. (1935). The basis of Ligon's theory. *American Journal of Psychology, 47*, 499–504.

Strub, R.L., & Black, F.W. (1977). *The mental status examination in neurology.* Philadelphia: F.A. Davis.

Strub, R.L., & Black, F.W. (1988). *Organic brain syndromes: An introduction to neurobehavioral disorders* (2nd ed.). Philadelphia: F.A. Davis.

Strub, R.L., & Black, F.W. (1993). *The mental status exam in neurology* (3rd ed.). Philadelphia: F.A. Davis.

Sunderland, T., Hill, J.L., Mellow, A.M., Lawlor, B.A., Gundersheimer, J., Newhouse, P.A., & Grafman, J.H. (1989). Clock drawing in Alzheimer's disease: A novel measure of dementia severity. *Journal of the American Geriatric Association, 37,* 725–729.

Sweet, J.J., Moberg, P.J., & Tovian, S.M. (1990). Evaluation of the Wechsler Adult Intelligence Scale-Revised premorbid IQ formulas in clinical populations. *Psychological Assessment, 2,* 41–44.

Taylor, R. (1982). *Mind or body: Distinguishing psychological from organic disorders.* New York: McGraw-Hill.

Teasdale, G., & Jennett, B. (1974). Assessment of coma and impaired consciousness. *The Lancet,* July 13, 1974, 81–83.

Terman, L.M., & Merrill, M.A. (1960). *Stanford-Binet Intelligence Scale: Manual for the third revision form L-M.* Boston: Houghton Mifflin.

Thurstone, L.L. (1938). *Primary mental abilities.* Chicago: University of Chicago Press.

Thurstone, L.L., & Thurstone, T.G. (1962). *Primary mental abilities* (rev. ed.). Chicago: Science Research Associates.

Tolor, A., & Schulberg, H. (1963). *An evaluation of the Bender-Gestalt.* Springfield, IL: Charles C. Thomas.

Tow, P.M. (1985). *Personality changes following frontal leucotomy.* New York: Oxford University Press.

Trauner, D.A. (1982). Seizure disorder. In W.G. Wiederholt (Ed.), *Neurology for non-neurologists* (pp. 283–297). New York: Academic Press.

Trimble, M.R., & Thompson, P.J. (1986). Neuropsychological aspects of epilepsy. In I. Grant & K.M. Adams (Eds.), *Neuropsychological assessment of neuropsychiatric disorders* (pp. 321–346). New York: Oxford University Press.

Tymchuk, A.J. (1974). Comparison of the Bender error and time scores from groups of epileptic, retarded, and behavior problem children. *Perceptual and Motor Skills, 38,* 71–79.

Tzavaras, A., Hecaen, H., & LeBras, H. (1970). Le probleme de la specificite du deficit de la reconnaissance du visage humain lors des lesions hemispheriques unilaterales. *Neuropsychologia, 8,* 403–416.

Vaughn, H.G., Jr., & Costa, L.D. (1962). Performance of patients with lateralized cerebral lesions: II. Sensory and motor tests. *Journal of Nervous and Mental Disease, 134,* 237–243.

Walsh, M.C., Groisser, D., & Pennington, B.F. (1988). *A normative-developmental study of performance on measures hypothesized to tap prefrontal functions.* Paper presented to the International Neuropsychological Society, New Orleans.

Wang, P.L. (1984). *Manual for the Modified Vygotsky Concept Formation Test.* Chicago: Stoelting.

Wang, P.L. (1990). Assessment of cognitive competency. In D.E. Tupper & K.D.

Cicerone (Eds.), *The neuropsychology of everyday life: Assessment and basic competencies*. Boston: Kluwer Academic Publishers.

Wang, P.L., & Ennis, K.E. (1986). Competency assessment in clinical populations: An introduction to the Cognitive Competency Test. In B. Uzzell & Y. Gross (Eds.), *Clinical neuropsychology of intervention*. Boston: Martinus Nijhoff.

Wang, P.L., Ennis, K., & Copeland, S. (1987). *Cognitive Competency Test*. Toronto: Mount Sinai Hospital, Psychology Department.

Warrington, E.K., & James, M. (1967). Disorders of visual perception in patients with localized cerebral lesions. *Neuropsychologia, 5*, 253–266.

Warrington, E.K., & Rabin, P. (1970). Perceptual matching in patients with cerebral lesions, *Neuropsychology, 8*, 475–487.

Watson, C.G. (1968). The separation of neuropsychiatric hospital organics from schizophrenics with three visual motor screening tests. *Journal of Clinical Psychology, 24*, 412–414.

Wechsler, D.A. (1945). A standardized memory scale for clinical use. *Journal of Psychology, 19*, 87–95.

Wechsler, D.A. (1981). *Manual for the Wechsler Adult Intelligence Scale-Revised*. New York: Psychological Corporation.

Wechsler, D. (1987). *Wechsler Memory Scale-Revised Manual*. San Antonio: The Psychological Corporation.

Wedding, D. (1986). Neurological disorders. In D. Wedding, A.M. Horton, Jr., & J. Webster (Eds.), *The neuropsychology handbook: Behavioral and clinical perspectives* (pp. 59–79). New York: Springer.

Wedding, D., Horton, A.M., Jr., & Webster, J. (1986). *The neuropsychology handbook: Behavioral and clinical perspectives*. New York: Springer.

Weigl, E. (1941). On the psychology of so-called processes of abstraction. *Journal of Abnormal and Social Psychology, 36*, 3–33.

Weinberger, D. (in press). *The neurology of schizophrenia*.

Weinstein, S. (1964). Deficits concomitant with aphasia or lesions of either cerebral hemisphere. *Cortex, 1*, 151–169.

Wells, C.E. (1979). Pseudodementia. *American Journal of Psychiatry, 136*, 895–900.

Wells, C.E., & Duncan, G.W. (1980). *Neurology for psychiatrists*. Philadelphia: F.A. Davis.

Wheeler, L., & Reitan, R. M. (1962). Presence and laterality of brain damage predicted from responses to a short aphasia screening test. *Perceptual and Motor Skills, 15*, 783–799.

Wheeler, L., & Reitan, R.M. (1963). Discriminant functions applied to the problem of predicting cerebral damage from behavioral testing: A cross-validation study. *Perceptual and Motor Skills, 16*, 681–701.

Wiederholt, W.C. (1982). Cerebrovascular disease. In W.C. Wiederholt (Ed.), *Neurology for non-neurologists* (pp. 179–189). New York: Academic Press.

Wiederholt, W.C. (1982). Dementias. In W.C. Wiederholt (Ed.), *Neurology for non-neurologists* (pp. 191–203). New York: Academic Press.

Wilkinson, G.S. (1993). *Wide Range Achievement Test 3*. Wilmington, DE: Jastak Associates.

Williams, J.M. (1991). *Memory Assessment Scales: Professional Manual.* Odessa, FL: Psychological Assessment Resources.

Wilson, B., Cockburn, J., & Baddeley, A. (1985). *The Rivermead Behavioural Memory Test.* Reading, United Kingdom: Thames Valley Test Company.

Wolf, J. K. (1980). *Practical clinical neurology.* Garden City, NY: Medical Examination Publishing.

Wolf-Klein, G.P., Silverstone, F.A., Levy, A.P., & Brod, M.S. (1989). Screening for Alzheimer's disease by clock drawing. *Journal of the American Psychiatric Association, 37*, 730–734.

Wolozin, B.L., Pruchnicki, A., Dickson, D.W., & Davies, P. (1986). A neuronal antigen in the brains of Alzheimer patients. *Science, 232*, 648–650.

Woodcock, R.W. (1973). *Woodcock Reading Mastery Tests.* Circle Pines, MN: American Guidance Service.

Wysocki, J.J., & Sweet, J.J. (1985). Identification of brain-damaged, schizophrenic, and normal medical patients using a brief neuropsychological screening battery. *International Journal of Clinical Neuropsychology, 7*, 40–44.

Yazdanfar, D.J. (1990). Assessing the mental status of the cognitively impaired elderly. *Journal of Gerontological Nursing, 16*, 32–36.

York Haaland, K., Vranes, L.F., Goodwin, J.S., & Garry, J.P. (1987). Wisconsin Card Sorting Test performance in a healthy elderly population. *Journal of Gerontology, 42*, 345–346.

Zangwill, O.L. (1966). Psychological deficits associated with frontal lobe lesions. *International Journal of Neurology, 5*, 395–402.

Zimet, C.N., & Fishman, D.B. (1970). Psychological deficit in schizophrenia and brain damage. *Annual Review of Psychology, 21*, 113–154.

Index

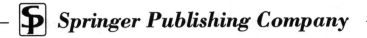

Springer Publishing Company

BIOSOCIAL PSYCHOPATHOLOGY

Epidemiological Perspectives

Donald I. Templer, PhD,
Dorothy A. Spencer, PhD, and
Lawrence C. Hartlage, PhD

The expert authors have created a seminal work that is further distinguished by its timely biosocial approach to the topic, which includes both neuropsychological and social aspects. This volume covers the full range of varied and complex problem behaviors, including schizophrenia, anxiety disorders, and eating disorders, among many others.

Contents:

I. Disorders of Brain Abnormality. Brain Disorders • Schizophrenia • Mental Retardation

II: Disorders of Subjective Experience. Anxiety Disorders • Mood Disorders • Sleep Disorders • Dissociative Disorders • Somatoform Disorders

III: Disorders of Self-Control. Disorders of Impulse Control • Eating Disorders • Alcoholism • Drug Abuse

IV: Disorders of Interpersonal Maladjustment. Personality Disorders • Sexual Disorders • Delusional (Paranoid) Disorders • Factitious Disorders

1994   344pp   0-8261-8290-9   hardcover

536 Broadway, New York, NY 10012-3955 • (212) 431-4370 • Fax (212) 941-7842

S *Springer Publishing Company*

SCREENING CHILDREN FOR BRAIN IMPAIRMENT

Michael D. Franzen, PhD
and **Richard Alan Berg**, PhD

"The thoroughness, clarity, scholarship, clinical relevance, and breadth of coverage of this clinical manual should make it a very popular clinical and reference tool for general clinicians and multidisciplinary specialists alike."

— **The American Psychological Assessment Exchange**

Contents:

General Disorders in Children and the Specialists Who Treat Them • Developmental Disorders • Neurological Disorders of Childhood • Psychiatric and Behavioral Disorders of Children • Neurological Soft Signs • The Interview and History • The Mental Status Exam in Children • The Wechsler Intelligence Scale for Children–Revised as a Screening Test of Perceptual, Cognitive, and Motor Functioning • The Kaufman Assessment Battery for Children • Screening Tests of Perceptual, Cognitive, and Motor Functioning • Verbal Screening Instruments • Screening Assessment of Very Young Children • The Differing Roles of Professional Specialties

Behavioral Science Book Service Selection
1989   272pp   0-8261-6390-4   softcover

536 Broadway, New York, NY 10012-3955 • (212) 431-4370 • Fax (212) 941-7842

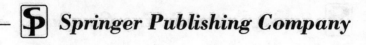
Springer Publishing Company

THE CLINICAL ASSESSMENT OF MEMORY
A Practical Guide

Dennis Reeves, PhD, and Danny Wedding, PhD

This quick and useful reference for the non-specialist clinician provides helpful guidelines for the administration and interpretation of carefully selected memory tests. The volume also provides a summary of current theories of memory, as well as a summary of the neuroanatomy of memory.

1993   240pp   0-8261-7920-1   hardcover

536 Broadway, New York, NY 10012-3955 • (212) 431-4370 • Fax (212) 941-7842